EMOTIONAL HEALER

Drop by Drop - Bach Flower Remedies

William Camolesi Di Biasi

As I share my thoughts with you, I would like, first of all, to make some clarifications. When I use the term "magic" in this book, I am not referring to the esoteric sense, but rather to what is often hidden from us, simply because we are not open to a good reading of the world. Another fact that should be observed is that in holistic therapies, nothing is quick and abrupt. We should always remember that we live in a world of urgencies, where everything is for yesterday, and when we feel discomfort or pain, we want an immediate solution, which we often only get through allopathy. What we must take into account is that energetic reprogramming takes a certain time, and unlike what we may hear out there, time is not faith. Being open to new forms of treatment has nothing to do with having faith in new treatments, it is just opening up to the possibility that even when it takes a little longer, the solution is coming.

This is my advice to anyone interested in holistic therapies: have patience, a little bit of calmness, and you will reach your goal. I know this is not easy, I also used to be part of this immediate movement, sometimes I still see myself in it. We live surrounded by an immense world, isn't it true, and we are also influenced by it.

Thinking like this, I would like to share the story I heard as a boy and that still helps me a lot today: "The Parable of the Scientist and the Child: How to Fix the World". For copyright reasons, I will not reproduce it here, but I advise reading it, but "spoiler" basically the child takes a cut-out of a map where there was a man on the back. Not knowing what the map was like, she turns the page and fixes the man. And when asked how she solved the puzzle so quickly, she gives the answer: "When I managed to fix the man, I turned the page and saw that I had fixed the world."

Sorry for that, but I warned you about the spoiler beforehand. I don't know the source of the story, I heard it as a child, read it a few times, but never knew the author.

And still in time, we must note the need not to close ourselves to what we do not know. Energetic healing is becoming more widely accepted by science, but it's still a new and uncharted territory for many. When I started my journey, I was considered by many as different, a little crazy, and other terms used in a not kind way. Today I see the same people seeking a new way of living, a better way of living. Give these topics a chance. Read, ask, research, see pros and cons and if you choose this path, be sure that you will be in good hands. At no time do I advise you to leave Western treatment or your doctor. I doubt that any therapist will give you a contrary advice.

I wish you luck, harmony, and good health on your journey.

As I sit down to write this introduction to Bach Flower Remedies, I can't help but feel a sense of excitement and wonder. What a beautiful and magical world we live in, where the healing powers of nature are at our fingertips!

In the following pages, we will explore the fascinating history and philosophy behind Bach Flower Remedies. We will delve into the intricate process of creating these remedies, and learn about the principles of vibrational healing that underpin their effectiveness.

But most importantly, we will discover how Bach Remedies can help us on our journey towards emotional and physical wellness. In today's fast-paced and often overwhelming world, it's more important than ever to find ways to take care of ourselves, and Bach Flower Remedies offer a gentle and holistic approach to achieving balance and harmony.

Whether you're struggling with anxiety or depression, grief or stress, or simply looking for ways to enhance your daily life, Bach Remedies have something to offer. With their natural and non-invasive approach, they are safe and accessible for everyone, and can be easily integrated into your daily routine.

So come along with me on this journey of discovery, and let's unlock the power of nature together. Let's explore the wonders of Bach Flower Remedies, and discover the joy and healing they can bring to our lives.

The history of Bach Flower Remedies is a fascinating journey that takes us back to the early 20th century, and the visionary work of Dr. Edward Bach. Born in 1886 in Birmingham, England, Dr. Bach was a highly respected physician and homeopath who dedicated his life to finding new and innovative ways to heal his patients.

It was during his time working in a London hospital that Dr. Bach began to notice a link between his patients' emotional states and their physical health. He believed that emotional imbalances and stress were major contributing factors to many illnesses, and that by addressing these underlying issues, he could help his patients achieve greater levels of health and well-being.

Inspired by the natural beauty of the English countryside, Dr. Bach began to explore the healing properties of flowers and plants. He believed that each plant had a unique energy and vibration, which could be harnessed to help restore balance to the mind and body.

Over the course of many years, Dr. Bach developed a system of 38 flower remedies, each one designed to address a specific emotional state or issue. He believed that by working with these remedies, patients could access their innate healing abilities and *overcome even the most stubborn physical and emotional challenges.*

Today, the legacy of Dr. Bach's work lives on, and his remedies are used by millions of people around the world. The popularity of Bach Flower Remedies has only grown in recent years, as more and more people seek out natural and holistic approaches to health and wellness.

As we delve deeper into the world of Bach Remedies, we will discover the many ways in which they can help us achieve greater levels of balance, harmony, and well-being. So, exploring the fascinating history of Bach Flower Remedies, we will uncover the secrets of their timeless healing power.

<u>The philosophy behind</u>

The philosophy behind Bach Flower Remedies is rooted in the idea that true healing comes from within. Dr. Edward Bach believed that the body has an innate ability to heal itself, and that by addressing the emotional and mental causes of illness, we can tap into this inner healing power.

According to Bach's philosophy, negative emotions such as fear, anxiety, and anger can disrupt the flow of energy in the body and lead to physical symptoms. By working with the vibrational energies of plants and flowers, Bach Remedies help to restore balance and harmony to the mind and body, allowing the body's natural healing processes to take over.

But the philosophy of Bach Remedies goes beyond just physical healing. It is rooted in the idea that emotional and mental well-being are essential components of overall health. By addressing emotional imbalances and negative thought patterns, Bach Remedies help to bring us back into alignment with our true selves and our higher purpose.

At the heart of Bach's philosophy is the belief that each of us has a unique path and purpose in life, and that by listening to our inner guidance and staying true to ourselves, we can achieve our fullest potential. Bach Remedies help us to tune into this inner guidance, and to overcome the fears and doubts that can hold us back from living our best lives.

The philosophy of Bach Remedies is simple yet profound, and it offers a powerful reminder of the healing power of nature and the importance of holistic approaches to health and wellness. As we explore the world of Bach Remedies, we will see how this philosophy is reflected in every aspect of these remedies, from their creation to their use in daily life.

How Bach Remedies are made

Have you ever wondered how Bach Remedies are made? The process is a fascinating and intricate one, rooted in the principles of vibrational healing and the wisdom of nature.

The first step in creating a Bach Remedy is to gather the flowers or plants that will be used. These plants are typically harvested at the peak of their vibrational energy, usually early in the morning when the sun is just rising.

Once the plants have been gathered, they are placed in a bowl of fresh spring water and left in the sun for several hours. This process allows the energy and vibration of the plant to infuse into the water, creating a potent vibrational remedy.

After the plant material has been removed, the resulting liquid is mixed with an equal amount of brandy to preserve the remedy and maintain its potency. This mixture is then bottled and labelled with the name of the flower or plant that was used.

It's important to note that the process of creating a Bach Remedy goes beyond just the physical aspects of the plants and the water. According to Bach's philosophy, the vibration and energy of the person who is creating the remedy is also an important factor.

This is why the process of creating Bach Remedies is done with great care and intention. The person creating the remedy must be in a calm and centred state, with a clear mind and a pure heart. This allows their own energy and vibration to be in harmony with the energy and vibration of the plant, creating a truly powerful healing remedy.

In conclusion, the process of creating Bach Remedies is a beautiful and intricate one, rooted in the principles of vibrational healing and the wisdom of nature. By harnessing the healing power of plants and flowers, Bach Remedies offer a gentle and holistic approach to achieving emotional and physical well-being, discovering the transformative power of nature in our lives.

To truly understand the power of Bach Remedies, we must first delve into the principles of vibrational healing. At its core, vibrational healing is based on the idea that everything in the universe, including our bodies, is made up of energy and vibration.

According to this principle, illness and emotional imbalance occur when the energy in our bodies becomes disrupted or blocked. Vibrational healing works by introducing new, harmonious frequencies into the body, which can help to clear blockages and restore balance to the body's energy field.

Bach Remedies are a form of vibrational healing that work by harnessing the energy and vibration of plants and flowers. Each plant or flower has its own unique energy signature, which can be used to address specific emotional imbalances or negative thought patterns.

For example, if someone is experiencing feelings of fear and anxiety, the Bach Remedy of Mimulus may be used. Mimulus is a flower that is associated with courage and inner strength, and its vibrational energy can help to dispel feelings of fear and promote confidence and self-assurance.

But how do these vibrational remedies work? The theory behind vibrational healing is that the energy and vibration of the remedy resonate with the energy and vibration of the person using it, helping to restore balance and harmony to their energy field.

While the principles of vibrational healing may seem esoteric or abstract, they are supported by a growing body of scientific research. Studies have shown that vibrational remedies can have a measurable impact on the body's energy field, and may help to promote feelings of calm and well-being.

In conclusion, understanding the principles of vibrational healing is key to unlocking the transformative power of Bach Remedies. By working with the energy and vibration of plants and flowers, these remedies offer a gentle and holistic approach to achieving emotional and physical well-being. So let us embrace the principles of vibrational healing, and discover the healing power of nature within ourselves.

Categories, Emotions – according with Dr. Bach

Dr. Bach approach to healing emphasized the importance of treating the root cause of an illness rather than just the symptoms. He believed that emotional imbalances were at the root of many physical ailments and that by addressing these emotional imbalances, true healing could occur.

So, he categorized emotions into 7 broad categories, which are still used today as a framework for understanding emotional imbalances and selecting appropriate Bach Flower Remedies.

Fear

Fear is a common and natural emotion, but when it becomes overwhelming and irrational, it can be debilitating. Fear can manifest in many forms, including fear of specific things, such as spiders or heights, or more general anxiety about the future.
Bach Flower Remedies for fear include Mimulus, Aspen, Cherry Plum, Red Chestnut, and Rock Rose. These remedies can help to alleviate feelings of fear and restore a sense of calm and courage.

Uncertainty

Uncertainty can be a difficult emotion to deal with, as it involves a sense of not knowing what the future holds. This can lead to indecision, doubt, and anxiety.

Bach Flower Remedies for uncertainty include Cerato, Scleranthus, Gentian, Gorse, and Hornbeam. These remedies can help to bring clarity, certainty, and a sense of direction.

Insufficient Interest in Present Circumstances

When we feel disconnected from the present moment, we may find ourselves constantly daydreaming or distracted. This can lead to feelings of dissatisfaction and restlessness.

Bach Flower Remedies for insufficient interest in present circumstances include Clematis, Honeysuckle, Wild Rose, Olive, and White Chestnut. These remedies can help us to stay grounded and engaged in the present moment.

Loneliness

Loneliness is a feeling of being isolated or disconnected from others. It can be a difficult emotion to deal with, as it can lead to feelings of sadness, despair, and low self-esteem.

Bach Flower Remedies for loneliness include Water Violet, Impatiens, Heather, Chicory, and Sweet Chestnut. These remedies can help us to connect with others and feel a sense of belonging.

Over-sensitivity to Influences and Ideas

When we are overly sensitive to the opinions of others or to the world around us, we can become easily overwhelmed and anxious.

Bach Flower Remedies for over-sensitivity include Agrimony, Centaury, Walnut, Holly, and Larch. These remedies can help us to stay centred and grounded, even in the face of external influences.

Despondency or Despair

Despondency or despair is a feeling of hopelessness and sadness that can be difficult to overcome. It can be a symptom of depression or other mental health issues.
Bach Flower Remedies for despondency or despair include Gentian, Gorse, Mustard, Sweet Chestnut, and Willow. These remedies can help to bring a sense of hope and optimism, even in difficult circumstances.

Over-care for Welfare of Others

When we become overly invested in the welfare of others, we can neglect our own needs and become exhausted or burned out.
Bach Flower Remedies for over-care include Chicory, Vervain, Vine, Beech, and Rock Water. These remedies can help us to set healthy boundaries and take care of ourselves, while still being compassionate towards others.

By understanding the 7 categories of emotions identified by Dr. Bach, we can gain insight into our own emotional imbalances and select appropriate Bach Flower Remedies to help us restore balance and harmony.

The 38 Bach Flower Remedies

Agrimony	Mimulus
Aspen	Mustard
Beech	Oak
Centaury	Olive
Cerato	Pine
Cherry Plum	Red Chestnut
Chestnut Bud	Rock Rose
Chicory	Rock Water
Clematis	Scleranthus
Crab Apple	Star of Bethlehem
Elm	Sweet Chestnut
Gentian	Vervain
Gorse	Vine
Heather	Walnut
Holly	Water Violet
Honeysuckle	White Chestnut
Hornbeam	Wild Oat
Impatiens	Wild Rose
Larch	Willow

Each of these remedies is associated with specific emotional states and can be used to help restore balance and harmony to the mind and body.

Now it's time to go deeper into each flower remedy. In the following chapters, I will try to explain each of the 38 remedies in a simplified way.

AGRIMONY

As I sat in the garden, surrounded by the soft fluttering of butterflies and the gentle rustling of leaves, I couldn't help but feel a sense of peace wash over me. It was in this moment that I realized the true power of Agrimony Bach Flower Remedy.

For those who may be unfamiliar, Agrimony is a gentle yet potent remedy that helps to ease inner turmoil and bring about a sense of calm. It's often used for those who put on a brave face in public but struggle with anxiety or inner conflict behind closed doors.

As I took my daily dose of Agrimony, I felt my mind become clearer and my thoughts more organized. The nagging worries and doubts that had been swirling around my head all day began to dissipate, leaving behind a sense of calm and tranquillity.

But what truly amazed me about Agrimony was its ability to help me confront and work through my inner demons. For years, I had been struggling with feelings of guilt and shame, but with Agrimony's help, I found the strength to confront these feelings head-on.

Through daily use of the remedy, I began to recognize the patterns and triggers that were causing my inner turmoil, and I was able to take steps towards healing and forgiveness. It wasn't easy, but with Agrimony's support, I was able to break free from the negative thought patterns that had been holding me back for so long.

And as I continued to use Agrimony, I found that it wasn't just my inner turmoil that was improving - my relationships with others were also benefiting. I was able to communicate more effectively, express my emotions more clearly, and establish deeper connections with those around me.

Agrimony Bach Flower Remedy has been a game-changer for me. It has helped me to find peace and clarity amidst the chaos of everyday life, and has given me the strength to confront my inner demons and grow as a person. I would highly recommend it to anyone who is struggling with anxiety, inner conflict, or feelings of guilt and shame.

<u>ASPEN</u>

The gentle rustling of leaves in the forest is soothing, but when the wind picks up and the trees start to creak and groan, it can be downright unnerving. For some people, this feeling of unease and anxiety isn't limited to the outdoors - it can creep into their everyday lives, causing them to feel on edge and fearful for no apparent reason. If this sounds like you, Aspen Bach Flower Remedy may be just what you need.

Aspen is a subtle yet powerful remedy that helps to ease feelings of anxiety and fear. Unlike some remedies that are tailored to specific situations or emotions, Aspen is a versatile remedy that can be used for a wide range of fears and anxieties.

The remarkable quality of Aspen that I appreciate the most is its ability to assist us in accessing our intuition and relying on our instincts. In many cases, we experience anxiety or fear because we sense subtle signs that we cannot quite comprehend. Aspen empowers us to trust our intuition and take action in a way that feels suitable for us.

Aside from easing anxiety, Aspen enables us to confront the unknown and gather the courage to leave our comfort zones. In times of fear or uncertainty, we tend to cling to what is familiar and avoid taking chances. But with the assistance of Aspen, we can summon the determination to take the initial steps towards novelty and adventure.

Of course, Aspen isn't a magic cure-all - like any remedy, it works best when used in conjunction with other healthy habits and self-care practices. But if you're looking for a gentle yet effective way to ease your anxiety and find the courage to take on new challenges, Aspen Bach Flower Remedy is definitely worth exploring.

In my own experience, Aspen has helped me to confront my fears and take on new challenges in both my personal and professional life. Whether it's speaking up in a meeting or trying a new hobby, I've found that Aspen gives me the extra boost of confidence and courage that I need to take those first steps. If you're ready to take control of your anxiety and find the courage to step outside of your comfort zone, I would definitely recommend giving Aspen a try.

<u>BEECH</u>

As human beings, we're wired to connect with others - to form friendships, build relationships, and work together towards common goals. But what happens when those connections break down? When we're constantly irritated or frustrated by the people around us, it can be difficult to maintain a sense of harmony and peace. That's where Beech Bach Flower Remedy comes in.

Beech is a powerful remedy that helps us to cultivate greater empathy and understanding towards others. Whether we're dealing with difficult coworkers, challenging family members, or just people who seem to rub us the wrong way, Beech can help us to soften our edges and see things from a different perspective.

One of the things that I love about Beech is its ability to help us recognize our own biases and assumptions. Often, when we're feeling irritated or frustrated by someone else's behaviour, it's because we're projecting our own insecurities or judgments onto them. But with Beech's help, we can take a step back and examine our own attitudes and beliefs, allowing us to approach the situation with greater clarity and compassion.

Of course, this isn't always easy - it can be difficult to let go of our own preconceived notions and see things from another person's point of view. But with Beech's gentle support, we can begin to break down those barriers and find common ground with those around us.

Another powerful aspect of Beech is its ability to foster greater tolerance and acceptance of differences. We live in a world that's full of diversity - of backgrounds, beliefs, and experiences - and it's all too easy to fall into the trap of judging others who don't share our own worldview. But with Beech's help, we can learn to celebrate those differences and appreciate the unique perspectives that others bring to the table.

In my own life, Beech has helped me to navigate difficult relationships and find greater harmony in my interactions with others. Whether I'm dealing with a frustrating coworker or a family member who seems to push my buttons, Beech has helped me to approach the situation with greater compassion and understanding. If you're looking for a way to cultivate greater empathy and acceptance towards those around you, I highly recommend considering the use of Beech Bach Flower Remedy.

<u>CENTAURY</u>

Do you find yourself constantly putting the needs of others before your own? Do you have a hard time saying no or setting boundaries, even when it comes at a cost to your own well-being? If so, you may benefit from Centaury Bach Flower Remedy.

Centaury is a powerful remedy that helps us to develop greater strength and independence. It's especially beneficial for those who struggle with codependency, feeling like they need to constantly cater to the needs of others in order to feel accepted or loved. With Centaury's support, we can learn to assert our own needs and boundaries, while still maintaining compassion and empathy towards others.

One of the things that I love about Centaury is its ability to help us break free from old patterns and habits. Often, those of us who struggle with codependency have learned these behaviours as a coping mechanism - a way to feel safe and accepted in a world that may not always feel supportive. But over time, these patterns can become deeply ingrained, making it difficult to even recognize when we're putting our own needs on the back burner.

Centaury helps us to step back and examine these patterns, allowing us to develop greater self-awareness and agency. With its support, we can learn to say no when we need to, set boundaries that protect our own well-being, and communicate our needs and desires with greater clarity and confidence.

Another powerful aspect of Centaury is its ability to help us develop a stronger sense of self-worth. When we're constantly putting the needs of others before our own, it can be difficult to even know what our own needs and desires are. But with Centaury's support, we can begin to cultivate a deeper understanding of our own value and worth, independent of the opinions or expectations of others.

In my own life, Centaury has been a valuable tool for developing greater self-care and self-compassion. By learning to recognize my own needs and set healthy boundaries, I've been able to cultivate a greater sense of balance and harmony in my relationships with others. If you struggle with codependency or find yourself constantly putting the needs of others before your own, I would definitely recommend giving Centaury Bach Flower Remedy a try.

<u>CERATO</u>

Are you someone who struggles with indecision or a lack of trust in your own intuition? Do you find yourself constantly seeking the advice and opinions of others, even when deep down you already know what you want or need? If so, Cerato Bach Flower Remedy may be just the remedy you need to help you tap into your inner wisdom and make decisions with greater confidence.

Cerato is a powerful remedy that helps to strengthen our connection to our own intuition and inner guidance. It's especially beneficial for those who struggle with self-doubt or have a tendency to second-guess themselves. With Cerato's support, we can learn to trust our own instincts and make decisions that are aligned with our highest good.

Cerato has an amazing ability to help us establish a deeper sense of self-awareness, which is something I find truly admirable. When we're indecisive or lack confidence in our own judgment, it's usually because we've become disconnected from our inner wisdom. We may have become overly reliant on external validation and opinions, causing us to lose sight of our own distinctive viewpoint.

Cerato helps us to reconnect with that inner wisdom, allowing us to tap into our own intuition and make decisions with greater clarity and confidence. With its support, we can learn to differentiate between our own inner voice and the opinions or expectations of others, making choices that are truly aligned with our own needs and desires.

Another powerful aspect of Cerato is its ability to help us develop greater self-trust. When we're constantly seeking the opinions and approval of others, it can be difficult to even know what our own preferences or desires are. But with Cerato's support, we can begin to cultivate a deeper sense of trust in ourselves, recognizing that we have the wisdom and insight to make the best decisions for our own lives.

Cerato has been a valuable tool for developing greater self-confidence and assertiveness. By learning to trust my own intuition and make decisions that are aligned with my own inner guidance, I've been able to step into my own power and create a life that truly feels authentic and fulfilling. If you struggle with indecision or lack of trust in yourself, I would highly recommend trying the Cerato Bach Flower Remedy if you are experiencing difficulties with indecision or lack of self-trust.

CHERRY PLUM

Cherry Plum Bach Flower Remedy is a powerful remedy that can help us manage intense emotions and impulses, particularly those that feel overwhelming or out of control. If you're someone who struggles with anxiety, anger, or fear, Cherry Plum may be just the remedy you need to find greater balance and inner peace.

One of the key benefits of Cherry Plum is its ability to help us regulate our emotions. When we're in the grip of intense emotions like anger or fear, it can be difficult to think clearly or make rational decisions. We may feel like we're losing control or that we're at the mercy of our emotions. Cherry Plum helps to calm those intense emotions and bring us back to a place of greater equilibrium.

Another powerful aspect of Cherry Plum is its ability to help us release our fears and anxieties. Often, when we're experiencing intense emotions, it's because we're afraid of something - perhaps we're afraid of being judged or rejected, or maybe we're afraid of the unknown. Cherry Plum helps us to confront and release those fears, allowing us to move through difficult emotions with greater ease and grace.

The potency of Cherry Plum lies in its ability to help us accept and embrace our own inner strength and resilience. During moments of distress or chaos, it is common to feel powerless or overwhelmed. However, Cherry Plum can help us access our innate emotional resources and find the courage to confront even the most daunting situations.

In my personal experience, Cherry Plum has been an invaluable remedy in managing anxiety and fear. By regulating my emotions and relinquishing my fears, I have been able to achieve a greater sense of calm and equilibrium in my life. Additionally, by embracing my own inner strength, I have been able to navigate challenging circumstances with greater confidence and resilience.

If you find yourself grappling with intense emotions or feelings of being out of control, Cherry Plum Bach Flower Remedy may be a viable solution to consider. With its support, you can learn to regulate your emotions, release your fears, and harness your own inner strength and resilience to face any situation that comes your way.

CHESTNUT BUD

Chestnut Bud is a Bach Flower Remedy that can be extremely helpful for those who feel stuck in repeating patterns of behaviour. This remedy is specifically targeted at helping individuals who have a hard time learning from their past mistakes and tend to repeat the same patterns over and over again.

If you find yourself making the same mistakes repeatedly, or if you feel as though you're not growing or learning from your experiences, Chestnut Bud may be the remedy for you. By working with this remedy, you can begin to break free from these patterns and open yourself up to new experiences and opportunities.

One of the key benefits of Chestnut Bud is its ability to help us gain greater self-awareness. When we're caught in repeating patterns of behaviour, it can be difficult to see things clearly and objectively. Chestnut Bud can help us to step back and view our experiences with fresh eyes, allowing us to see where we may be making the same mistakes repeatedly.

Another benefit of Chestnut Bud is that it can help us to develop greater mindfulness. By becoming more present and aware of our thoughts, feelings, and behaviours, we can begin to notice when we're slipping into old patterns and make a conscious effort to change course.

If you're interested in working with Chestnut Bud, it's important to remember that this remedy won't magically solve all of your problems overnight. It's a tool that can help you to develop greater self-awareness and mindfulness, but ultimately, the work of breaking free from old patterns and creating new ones is up to you.

To get the most out of Chestnut Bud, it can be helpful to pair it with other healing modalities such as therapy or mindfulness practices like meditation or yoga. By combining different tools and techniques, you can create a holistic approach to healing and personal growth.

In conclusion, if you find yourself repeating the same patterns of behaviour and struggling to learn from your experiences, Chestnut Bud may be the Bach Flower Remedy for you. By working with this remedy and incorporating other healing modalities, you can break free from old patterns and create a life that feels more authentic and fulfilling.

CHICORY

Chicory Bach Flower Remedy can help those who struggle with over-attachment and possessiveness in their relationships. This remedy can aid in developing a stronger sense of inner security and promoting a more selfless way of loving.

One significant benefit of Chicory is its ability to assist us in relinquishing the need for control in relationships. When we become too attached and possessive, it can be challenging to find a way out. Chicory can help us let go of these feelings and foster a sense of inner security, allowing us to love more freely and selflessly.

Another remarkable aspect of Chicory is its ability to help us cultivate a compassionate and understanding attitude towards others. Feelings of possessiveness can often lead to demands and criticism of our loved ones. Chicory can help us adopt a more compassionate outlook, enabling us to approach our relationships with more kindness and understanding.

However, the most notable advantage of Chicory is its capacity to help us develop a greater sense of self-love and self-acceptance. When we become possessive and over-attached, we often seek validation and love from others. Chicory can help us appreciate our own worth and value, allowing us to love ourselves fully and deeply.

In my personal experience, Chicory has been an invaluable tool in cultivating healthier and more fulfilling relationships. By releasing the need for control and adopting a more compassionate approach, I've been able to form deeper connections and experience more love and fulfilment.

If you're struggling with possessiveness or over-attachment in your relationships, I highly recommend giving Chicory Bach Flower Remedy a chance. With its support, you can develop a stronger sense of inner security, approach your relationships with greater compassion and understanding, and learn to love yourself more fully and deeply, resulting in healthier and more fulfilling relationships.

<u>CLEMATIS</u>

Clematis is one of the most well-known Bach Flower Remedies, and it is often recommended for those who are struggling with feelings of detachment or disconnection from the present moment. If you find yourself constantly daydreaming or fantasizing about a different reality, Clematis may be the perfect remedy to help bring you back down to earth.

At its core, Clematis is about bringing a sense of clarity and focus to the mind. When we're caught up in our daydreams or fantasies, we're not fully present in the moment, which can make it difficult to make decisions or take action towards our goals. Clematis can help to ground us in the present moment, allowing us to see things more clearly and make decisions with greater confidence.

Clematis possesses the fascinating quality of allowing us to access our innate creativity. While daydreaming, we tend to explore novel ideas and concepts that we may not have otherwise considered. Through the use of Clematis, we can channel this creative energy and utilize it to facilitate our own individual progress and advancement.

Clematis is also a remedy that is often recommended for those who are dealing with physical or emotional pain. When we're in pain, it's easy to retreat into our own minds and escape into our daydreams as a way of coping. However, this can prevent us from fully addressing the root cause of our pain and finding the healing that we need. Clematis can help to bring us back into the present moment and allow us to fully process our emotions and physical sensations, leading to greater healing and self-awareness.

One of the things that I love about Clematis is how versatile it is as a remedy. Whether you're struggling with feelings of detachment or disconnection, or you simply need help focusing and staying present in the moment, Clematis can be a valuable tool in your healing journey.

If you're considering trying Clematis, it's important to remember that Bach Flower Remedies are not a one-size-fits-all solution. It's important to take the time to really tune into your own unique needs and intentions before selecting a remedy. As always, if you're uncertain which remedy might be right for you, it's a good idea to consult with a Bach Flower Practitioner or other qualified health professional who can provide guidance and support.

CRAB APPLE

Crab Apple Bach Flower Remedy is one of the most versatile remedies in the Bach Flower system, and is known for its ability to promote purity and cleanliness, both physically and mentally.

Physically, Crab Apple is often used to address skin conditions or other physical ailments that are related to feelings of uncleanliness or self-disgust. It can also be used to support the body's natural detoxification process, helping to eliminate toxins and restore balance.

Mentally, Crab Apple is often used to address feelings of self-consciousness or shame, particularly around issues of cleanliness or physical appearance. It can help to release feelings of self-disgust and promote a sense of inner purity and self-acceptance.

In addition to its physical and mental benefits, Crab Apple is also known for its spiritual properties. It is often used to promote a sense of inner clarity and alignment with one's higher self, helping to release negative thoughts and emotions that can cloud our spiritual vision.

One of the key ways in which Crab Apple can be used is by incorporating it into a daily self-care practice. This might involve adding a few drops of the remedy to a bath or foot soak, or applying it topically to the skin. Alternatively, it can be taken internally as a tincture or in a diluted form.

Another way to work with Crab Apple is through its energetic properties. Simply holding the remedy in your hand or meditating with it can help to align your energy and promote feelings of inner purity and self-acceptance.

Crab Apple can also be used in combination with other Bach Flower Remedies to address specific emotional issues or challenges. For example, it might be combined with Impatiens to promote a sense of calm and patience, or with Rock Rose to address feelings of extreme fear or panic.

In my own life, I have found Crab Apple to be a valuable tool for promoting physical and mental purity. By incorporating it into my self-care routine and working with its energetic properties, I have been able to release feelings of self-disgust and promote a sense of inner cleanliness and self-acceptance.

If you struggle with feelings of uncleanliness, self-consciousness, or shame, I would definitely recommend giving Crab Apple Bach Flower Remedy a try. With its support, you can learn to promote physical and mental purity, align with your higher self, and release negative thoughts and emotions that may be holding you back.

Elm is a Bach Flower Remedy that is particularly beneficial for people who are typically confident and capable but may occasionally find themselves feeling overwhelmed or struggling with their responsibilities. This remedy is often referred to as the "temporary loss of confidence" remedy and can provide relief to individuals who are normally able to handle their responsibilities with ease but are currently feeling overwhelmed.

Elm Bach Flower Remedy can provide particular assistance to those who hold positions of authority, such as managers or leaders, and suddenly experience difficulty in handling their responsibilities. This can result in significant anxiety and stress, but Elm can help to alleviate these emotions and restore confidence and calmness.

Furthermore, Elm can be beneficial for individuals who are taking on new challenges or projects and may be feeling uncertain about their abilities. This remedy can instil the necessary confidence to succeed and prevent feelings of being overwhelmed.

Elm can also be advantageous in relieving physical symptoms related to stress and anxiety, such as headaches or digestive issues. By addressing these physical symptoms, Elm can contribute to an overall improvement in wellbeing.
It's important to note that Elm is not a remedy for chronic lack of confidence or ongoing feelings of overwhelm. It is specifically

designed to address temporary feelings of anxiety and stress that are related to specific situations or responsibilities.

When using Elm, it's crucial to follow the instructions for preparation and use carefully. It's essential to seek the guidance of a qualified practitioner when using any Bach Flower Remedy.

In conclusion, Elm is a valuable tool for individuals who are typically confident and capable but occasionally find themselves feeling overwhelmed or struggling with their responsibilities. By helping to restore confidence and alleviate stress and anxiety, Elm can help individuals to feel more capable and able to handle their responsibilities with ease.

GENTIAN

Gentian is a Bach flower remedy that can help those who have lost faith and optimism due to a setback or disappointment. It's for those who find it hard to bounce back from negative experiences and may feel stuck in a cycle of negativity and pessimism.

At times, life can throw us unexpected challenges and setbacks that can be difficult to overcome. When we face such situations, it's common to feel disheartened, demotivated and lose hope. In these times, the Gentian Bach flower remedy can be a valuable tool to help us regain faith in ourselves and the world.

The Gentian remedy is particularly helpful for people who tend to dwell on the negative and have a hard time seeing the good in situations. These individuals may struggle to move forward, as they find it challenging to believe in themselves or that things will get better. They may also have a tendency to give up easily, feeling that their efforts are futile.

When we take Gentian, it helps us to see the silver lining in situations and to trust that everything happens for a reason. We begin to develop a more positive outlook, which allows us to move forward with hope and confidence. This newfound sense of positivity can also help us to feel more motivated and productive, as we are no longer bogged down by negative thoughts and feelings.

One of the best things about the Gentian remedy is that it can help us break free from the cycle of negativity. When we begin to see the good in situations, we naturally attract more positivity into our lives. As a result, we start to feel more fulfilled, happy, and content.

If you are struggling with setbacks and find it hard to maintain a positive outlook, taking the Gentian Bach flower remedy may be helpful. It can be especially useful during times of change, such as starting a new job, moving to a new place, or going through a breakup. By helping you to maintain a positive outlook, Gentian can help you navigate these transitions with more ease and grace.

Gentian Bach flower remedy is a powerful tool for anyone struggling with feelings of hopelessness and pessimism. By helping to restore faith in oneself and the world, it allows us to move forward with hope and confidence. If you're feeling stuck in a cycle of negativity, consider giving Gentian a try and see the positive changes it can bring to your life.

GORSE

If you're experiencing a sense of hopelessness or despair, Gorse may be the remedy for you. This flower essence helps to bring light back into our lives when we feel like we're stuck in a dark place. Gorse is especially helpful for those who have given up hope of finding a solution to their problems and have resigned themselves to a life of sadness or suffering.

Gorse is a bright yellow flowering plant that grows in the wild. It is often associated with the sun and brings a sense of warmth and positivity to those who use it. The Gorse Bach Flower Remedy is made by infusing the flowers of this plant in spring water and brandy.

When we feel hopeless or despairing, it's easy to get stuck in a negative mindset. We may start to believe that things will never get better and that there's no point in trying. Gorse helps to break this cycle of negativity by giving us a renewed sense of hope and positivity.

With Gorse, we can begin to see the possibilities that exist in our lives, even in the face of difficult circumstances. We can start to believe that things can get better, and that we have the strength and resilience to overcome our challenges.

Gorse is especially useful for those who have been through a prolonged period of suffering or adversity. It can be difficult to *find hope when we've been struggling for a long time, but Gorse helps us to see that there is still a light at the end of the tunnel.*

When we feel hopeless or despairing, it's important to remember that we're not alone. There are always people who care about us and want to help us through difficult times. Gorse can help us to connect with these sources of support and to open ourselves up to new possibilities.

If you're feeling stuck in a negative mindset, Gorse may be the remedy you need to bring light back into your life. With this flower essence, you can find hope and positivity, even in the darkest of times. So don't give up hope – try Gorse today and see how it can help you to find your way back to a happier and more fulfilling life.

HEATHER

Heather Bach Flower Remedy is one of the most popular remedies in the Bach Flower system. It is used to treat people who are excessively talkative, self-centred and need constant attention from others. They tend to dominate conversations, interrupting others and not allowing them to speak. They often feel lonely and isolated because their behaviour drives people away from them.

The remedy is made from the flowers of the Heather plant, which grows in the heathlands of Scotland. The plant itself is a hardy evergreen shrub that can survive in harsh and inhospitable environments. The flowers are small and bell-shaped, and they bloom in the summer months. The essence of the flowers is used to create the remedy.

Heather is recommended for people who are unable to be alone and need constant company. They are afraid of being by themselves, and so they seek the company of others all the time. They may appear to be outgoing and sociable, but this is just a mask to hide their true feelings of loneliness and despair.

By calming the mind and reducing anxiety, Heather Bach Flower Remedy facilitates self-awareness and introspection, leading to a restored sense of balance and harmony that allows for a more objective perspective. With decreased self-centeredness and increased empathy, individuals become more supportive of others, fostering stronger relationships.

A crucial lesson from Heather is the importance of self-love and acceptance in order to extend those qualities to others. When one finds inner peace and contentment, the need for validation and attention from others diminishes, leading to greater self-reliance and independence, and thus deeper and more meaningful relationships with others.

Heather is a gentle and safe remedy suitable for anyone, regardless of age or gender. It is available in various forms, including drops, sprays, and pills, and can be taken orally or applied topically as preferred.

In summary, Heather Bach Flower Remedy is a potent tool for self-discovery and personal growth, promoting self-awareness and self-acceptance essential to healthy relationships with others. It is a valuable addition to any self-care regimen and can help individuals overcome fears and anxieties, enabling them to live more fulfilling and satisfying lives.

Holly Bach Flower Remedy is a life-changing remedy that can help us break free from the grip of negative emotions such as hatred, jealousy, and anger. These emotions can be incredibly destructive, leading to even more negative thoughts and actions if left unchecked.

The beauty of Holly Bach Flower Remedy is that it helps us transform these negative emotions into positive ones, such as love and compassion. This powerful remedy enables us to address the root causes of our negative emotions and begin the journey towards personal transformation.

By taking Holly Bach Flower Remedy, we can cultivate feelings of love and compassion towards others, even in the face of anger or hatred. It helps us shift our perspective and see others in a more positive light, fostering a sense of connection and empathy.

Moreover, Holly Bach Flower Remedy can help us deal with jealousy, an emotion that often stems from feelings of inadequacy or a sense of not being good enough. By taking Holly, we can start to address these underlying issues and cultivate a sense of self-love and acceptance, leading to a more positive outlook on life.

This remedy can also shield us from external triggers that can cause negative emotions, such as exposure to news stories filled with hate and anger. By taking Holly, we can maintain a sense of inner peace, even in the face of adversity.

Lastly, Holly Bach Flower Remedy can be incredibly helpful during times of grief and loss, as it helps us process our emotions in a healthy way and move towards a state of acceptance and peace.

Overall, Holly Bach Flower Remedy is a powerful tool for personal growth and transformation. It helps us break free from the cycle of negative emotions and cultivate a sense of love, compassion, and positivity towards ourselves and others.

Discovering one's emotional blockages and finding ways to release them is essential to achieving inner peace and happiness. For those who struggle with being emotionally stuck in the past, Honeysuckle Bach Flower Remedy is here to help. This remedy, which is one of the 38 remedies developed by Dr. Edward Bach, is designed to free individuals from old memories and experiences that hold them back from enjoying the present.

The sweet-smelling, yellow-white flowers of Honeysuckle, a climbing vine that grows in temperate regions of the world, are used to create the flower essence used in Bach Flower Therapy. This remedy is particularly effective for those who suffer from nostalgia, regret, and an inability to move on from the past. It is not uncommon for these individuals to feel attached to people, situations, or habits that no longer serve them, which can prevent them from embracing the present and moving forward with their lives.

By using Honeysuckle Bach Flower Remedy, these individuals can let go of emotional attachments to the past and start living in the present. The remedy helps individuals break free from the emotional chains that hold them back and enables them to focus on the joys of the present. It is particularly helpful during times of transition, such as moving to a new city or starting a new job.

Honeysuckle is a potent remedy that can help individuals find closure and move on from the past. It encourages them to live in the present and look forward to the future with optimism and hope. Whether used alone or in combination with other Bach Flower Remedies, Honeysuckle Bach Flower Remedy can help treat a range of emotional imbalances.

If you find yourself struggling with feelings of nostalgia or regret that hold you back from enjoying the present, Honeysuckle Bach Flower Remedy can help. It can help you release the emotional chains of the past and start living in the present with an open heart and a positive outlook.

HORNBEAM

Hornbeam Bach Flower Remedy could be the solution for you if you experience a sense of weariness and exhaustion, both mentally and physically, but still manage to carry out your daily tasks.

This Bach Flower Remedy is specifically designed for those who experience a "Monday morning feeling" or a general sense of weariness and lack of motivation. But don't worry, Hornbeam can help you overcome these feelings and bring renewed energy and enthusiasm into your life. It can help you tackle overwhelming or uninteresting tasks with ease and confidence.

Hornbeam promotes mental clarity and focus, helping you overcome procrastination and become more productive. You may feel overwhelmed when starting tasks, but once you begin, you'll find the motivation to keep going. Hornbeam clears the foggy feeling in your mind and brings a sense of mental alertness.

If you're feeling emotionally drained or disconnected from the world around you, Hornbeam can help. This remedy reconnects you with your emotions and the world around you, helping you find joy and enthusiasm for life. By promoting emotional well-being, Hornbeam can help you feel more confident, connected, and engaged with the world.

Hornbeam is a gentle remedy that can be used in combination with other natural remedies or therapies to support emotional well-being. It's completely safe and non-toxic, making it an ideal choice for anyone seeking natural and non-invasive healing methods.

In summary, Hornbeam Bach Flower Remedy is a powerful tool for emotional healing, specifically designed for those who experience weariness and lack of motivation. It promotes mental clarity and focus, helps you overcome procrastination, and supports emotional well-being. With renewed energy and enthusiasm, Hornbeam can help you achieve overall health and well-being.

IMPATIENS

Impatiens Bach Flower Remedy is the perfect solution for those who struggle with impatience. If you are someone who is constantly in a hurry, easily frustrated by delays, and struggles to work with others, then Impatiens might be the remedy you need to help you achieve a greater sense of calm and inner peace.

The Impatiens flower is characterized by its bright purple colour and delicate, trumpet-shaped blooms. It grows in moist, shady areas, and can often be found near streams and rivers. According to Dr. Bach, the Impatiens flower embodies the qualities of patience, tolerance, and understanding, and can be used to help those who struggle with impatience to find greater balance and harmony in their lives.

When taken as a Bach Flower Remedy, Impatiens can help to calm the mind, reduce anxiety, and promote a greater sense of inner peace. It can also help to promote empathy and understanding towards others, making it easier to work with colleagues and family members, and reducing the stress and tension that can come from feeling constantly rushed and frustrated.

One of the most powerful benefits of Impatiens is that it can help to bring a sense of balance to your life. When you are constantly in a rush, it can be easy to become overwhelmed and stressed, leading to a sense of burnout and exhaustion. Impatiens can help to reduce these feelings, allowing you to approach life with a greater sense of calm and clarity.

If you are struggling with impatience, taking Impatiens as a Bach Flower Remedy can be an effective way to bring greater balance to your life. By promoting patience, tolerance, and understanding, Impatiens can help you to find greater peace and harmony, allowing you to work more effectively with others and achieve your goals with greater ease.

Impatiens Bach Flower Remedy is an effective solution for those who struggle with impatience. By promoting patience, tolerance, and understanding, Impatiens can help to reduce stress, anxiety, and tension, allowing you to approach life with a greater sense of calm and clarity. So, if you're struggling with impatience, consider trying Impatiens Bach Flower Remedy today, and see how it can help you to achieve greater balance and harmony in your life.

<u>LARCH</u>

Are you someone who struggles with self-doubt and a lack of self-esteem? Do you find yourself frequently holding back, hesitant to take risks or pursue your goals? If so, you may benefit from the Larch Bach Flower Remedy.

The Larch remedy is designed to help those who lack confidence in their abilities, often due to past failures or negative experiences. This remedy can be particularly useful for those who have a fear of failure, and therefore avoid trying new things or taking on challenges.

When taken as directed, Larch can help to promote a sense of self-assurance and courage, allowing individuals to approach new situations with greater confidence and ease. This remedy can be especially beneficial for those who struggle in social or professional situations, as it can help to alleviate anxiety and self-doubt.

The Larch remedy is made from the flowers of the Larch tree, which is known for its resilience and strength. By harnessing the natural properties of this tree, the Larch remedy can help to strengthen and fortify an individual's sense of self-worth and self-belief.

When taking the Larch remedy, it's important to remember that it is not a magic cure for all of life's challenges. Rather, it is a tool that can help to support and empower individuals as they navigate their own unique journey.

It's also important to note that the Larch remedy is not intended to replace professional therapy or medical treatment. Rather, it can be used in conjunction with other forms of support to help individuals overcome their self-doubt and build a stronger sense of self-confidence.

So if you're someone who struggles with a lack of self-esteem or confidence, consider giving the Larch Bach Flower Remedy a try. With its natural and gentle approach, it may be just the tool you need to unlock your true potential and achieve your goals with confidence and grace.

MIMULUS

Mimulus is a Bach Flower Remedy that is commonly used to help alleviate fear and anxiousness in individuals. It is derived from the Mimulus plant, a delicate flower that grows in damp conditions along streams and riverbanks.

The Mimulus flower is known for its vibrant yellow petals and delicate beauty, and it has been used for centuries to treat a variety of ailments. In the context of Bach Flower Remedies, Mimulus is specifically targeted towards individuals who are struggling with a specific, identifiable fear or anxiety.

People who may benefit from the Mimulus remedy include those who experience anxiety or nervousness before public speaking, or those who have a fear of spiders, heights, or enclosed spaces. These fears may be specific and easily identifiable, or they may be more general and undefined.

The Mimulus remedy works by addressing the underlying emotions that contribute to these fears and anxieties. By tapping into the vibrational energy of the Mimulus flower, individuals are able to restore a sense of calm and peace to their lives, even in the face of their fears.

The Mimulus remedy is particularly effective when used as part of a holistic treatment plan that includes therapy, lifestyle changes, and other natural remedies. It can be taken orally, applied topically, or even used in aromatherapy, depending on the individual's preferences and needs.

One of the key benefits of Mimulus Bach Flower Remedy is its ability to help individuals overcome their fears in a gentle and non-invasive way. Unlike traditional medications or therapies, which may have negative side effects or require significant lifestyle changes, Mimulus works by tapping into the body's natural ability to heal itself.

Another benefit of Mimulus is its accessibility. As a natural remedy, it is safe and non-toxic, making it an ideal choice for individuals who are seeking alternatives to traditional medications or therapies. It can be used by individuals of all ages, and is particularly beneficial for children who may be struggling with anxiety or nervousness.

In conclusion, Mimulus Bach Flower Remedy is a powerful and effective tool for individuals who are struggling with fear and anxiousness. By tapping into the healing power of the Mimulus flower, individuals are able to overcome their fears in a gentle and non-invasive way. Whether used as part of a holistic treatment plan or on its own, Mimulus has the potential to transform lives and restore a sense of calm and peace to individuals who are struggling with anxiety and fear.

<h1 style="text-align:center;"><u>MUSTARD</u></h1>

Mustard Bach Flower Remedy is one of the most interesting and unique remedies in the Bach system. This remedy is derived from the wild mustard plant, and it is known for its ability to alleviate the feelings of deep, unexplainable sadness and depression. If you are experiencing feelings of despair, gloom, or melancholy that seem to come out of nowhere, Mustard might be the right remedy for you.

Unlike other remedies that focus on a specific emotion or situation, Mustard is often recommended for people who experience depressive feelings without an apparent cause. In fact, the Mustard remedy is sometimes called the "black cloud" remedy because it describes the sudden onset of a dark and heavy mood that seems to hang over a person like a cloud.

One of the most fascinating things about the Mustard remedy is that it has no rational explanation for its effects. It does not work by directly targeting any specific physical or emotional ailment. Instead, it seems to work on a subtle level, re-establishing a person's emotional balance and helping them to regain their inner sense of peace and harmony.

Another unique aspect of the Mustard remedy is that it is an example of vibrational healing. This means that the remedy works not by its chemical composition, but by the subtle energy pattern it carries. In other words, the energy of the Mustard plant is imprinted onto the water used to make the remedy, and this energy is then transferred to the person who takes it.

If you are drawn to the Mustard remedy, it is important to note that it is not a quick fix. While some people experience an immediate improvement in their mood after taking the remedy, others may take several days or even weeks to see the full effects. It is also important to note that the Mustard remedy is not a substitute for professional medical advice or treatment.

In conclusion, the Mustard is a unique and fascinating remedy that has helped many people to overcome feelings of deep sadness and depression. It is a gentle and holistic approach to emotional wellness that focuses on restoring balance and harmony to the inner self. If you are experiencing feelings of unexplainable sadness or depression, the Mustard remedy might be the right choice for you.

OAK

Oak Bach Flower Remedy is a powerful essence that helps individuals find inner strength and resilience during tough times. This remedy is especially helpful for those who are driven and determined but may push themselves too hard and neglect their own needs.

If you are someone who often finds yourself tirelessly working towards your goals, even at the cost of your own wellbeing, Oak can offer you the support you need to maintain balance and harmony in your life. The essence of this flower helps individuals develop a healthy sense of self-awareness, enabling them to recognize when they need to rest and recharge.

Oak Bach Flower Remedy can also help individuals break free from patterns of stubbornness or inflexibility. Sometimes, in our pursuit of excellence and success, we become rigid and unwilling to change. Oak helps individuals find a healthy balance between determination and adaptability, allowing them to pursue their goals while remaining open to new ideas and experiences.

The essence of Oak is particularly helpful for those who experience burnout, whether due to work-related stress or other sources of pressure. It can help individuals build resilience, allowing them to maintain their focus and energy even during challenging times. Oak can also help individuals find a sense of peace and calmness amidst chaos, allowing them to handle unexpected situations with grace and ease.

While Oak is a powerful essence, it is important to remember that it is not a magic solution to all of life's problems. It is merely a tool that can help individuals develop a healthier relationship with themselves and the world around them. The true power of Oak lies in its ability to help individuals tap into their inner strength and resilience, allowing them to overcome obstacles and live their best lives.

If you are considering trying Oak Bach Flower Remedy, it is important to do so under the guidance of a qualified practitioner. They can help you develop a personalized treatment plan that addresses your unique needs and goals. With their support and the power of Oak, you can find the strength and resilience you need to thrive in today's fast-paced world.

<u>*OLIVE*</u>

Olive is a Bach Flower Remedy that is derived from the Olive tree, an evergreen symbol of peace and renewal. This remedy is intended to alleviate exhaustion, both mental and physical, and to provide the user with a sense of renewed energy and vitality. The Olive tree has been a symbol of peace, strength, and longevity for centuries, and the Olive Bach Flower Remedy aims to imbue its users with those same qualities.

Olive is a remedy that is particularly useful for those who have experienced burnout or fatigue, whether from work, personal life, or other sources of stress. It can help those who feel drained, depleted, or overwhelmed to find the strength and energy to carry on. This remedy works by stimulating the body's natural healing processes, promoting a sense of renewal and rejuvenation.

When using Olive, it is important to remember that this remedy is not a quick fix. It is not intended to provide an instant burst of energy or to mask underlying issues. Rather, it is a tool for promoting long-term renewal and rejuvenation. Olive can be used in conjunction with other Bach Flower Remedies to address specific issues, or it can be used on its own as a general tonic for exhaustion.

One of the unique aspects of Olive is that it works on both physical and mental exhaustion. This is because physical and mental exhaustion are often intertwined. When we are physically exhausted, our mental energy is also depleted, and vice versa. OLIVE can help to break this cycle by promoting a sense of overall renewal and vitality.

The benefits of Olive are numerous. It can help to restore balance to the body and mind, promoting a sense of overall well-being. It can also help to improve mental clarity and focus, which can be particularly useful for those who are feeling overwhelmed or burned out. Additionally, Olive can help to reduce feelings of stress and anxiety, which are often associated with exhaustion.

If you are feeling exhausted or burned out, Olive may be the right Bach Flower Remedy for you. It is a gentle and natural way to promote renewal and rejuvenation, and can be used in conjunction with other remedies to address specific issues. Whether you are looking to restore balance to your body and mind, improve your mental clarity and focus, or simply reduce feelings of stress and anxiety, Olive can help you on your journey towards renewed energy and vitality.

<u>PINE</u>

Specifically designed to address feelings of guilt and self-blame. Those who would benefit from this remedy are individuals who have a tendency to be hard on themselves, who blame themselves for mistakes or misfortunes, and who have a sense of not deserving happiness or good things in life.

Pine essence works by helping individuals to gain a more balanced and compassionate perspective on themselves. It helps to promote a more positive self-image, where one can recognize their strengths and accept their flaws without judgment. It also helps to cultivate a more forgiving attitude towards oneself, acknowledging that everyone makes mistakes and that these mistakes are part of the learning process.

One of the key indications for Pine remedy is the feeling of guilt or shame. This could be in response to a specific event or circumstance, or it could be a general feeling of inadequacy. Individuals who need Pine remedy often apologize excessively, even for things that are not their fault, and tend to take on responsibility for things that are outside of their control.

In addition to guilt and self-blame, Pine remedy can also help individuals who have a sense of unworthiness or self-punishment. This may manifest as a tendency to take on more work than one can handle, to avoid rest or leisure activities, or to put oneself in harm's way unnecessarily. Pine remedy can help individuals to recognize their own limits and to find a healthy balance between work and relaxation.

Another indication for Pine remedy is a lack of self-confidence. Individuals who need this remedy often doubt their own abilities, even in situations where they are competent and skilled. They may avoid taking on new challenges or responsibilities because of fear of failure or fear of being judged by others. Pine remedy can help individuals to overcome these feelings of inadequacy and to develop a more positive self-image.

Pine is a helpful tool for those who struggle with feelings of guilt, self-blame, and unworthiness. By promoting self-acceptance, forgiveness, and a more balanced perspective, Pine remedy can help individuals to live a more fulfilling and confident life.

RED CHESTNUT

If you tend to worry about others excessively, often experiencing anxiety for their safety and well-being, you might benefit from the Red Chestnut Bach Flower Remedy. This remedy is specifically designed to help individuals who have a tendency to overprotect their loved ones, often at the expense of their own emotional and physical health.

If you find yourself constantly fretting about your children, spouse, or close friends, fearing for their safety or well-being, Red Chestnut can help. This remedy works by restoring a sense of trust and faith in the natural course of events, allowing you to let go of the need to control and protect others.

By taking Red Chestnut, you can learn to balance your concern for others with a healthy dose of detachment and perspective. You can still care deeply for your loved ones, but without the constant worry and fear that can lead to stress, anxiety, and even physical symptoms.

The Red Chestnut remedy is especially useful for parents who struggle with overprotectiveness towards their children. If you find yourself constantly worrying about your children's safety, health, or happiness, you might be inadvertently transmitting your fears and anxieties onto them. By taking Red Chestnut, you can learn to trust in your children's ability to cope with life's challenges, and to let them develop their own sense of resilience and independence.

Furthermore, Red Chestnut can help those who work in caring professions, such as healthcare providers, social workers, or teachers. These individuals may experience a heightened sense of empathy and concern for their patients or students, often to the point of exhaustion and burnout. By taking Red Chestnut, they can learn to maintain a healthy distance and perspective, while still providing compassionate care and support.

In conclusion, Red Chestnut can be a helpful remedy for individuals who experience difficulties with empathy and overprotectiveness. It can support in the restoration of trust and belief in the natural flow of life events, aiding individuals in overcoming their worries and concerns, and fostering a well-adjusted approach towards looking after their loved ones. Whether an individual is a parent, caregiver, or someone who cares deeply for others, Red Chestnut remedy can assist in finding emotional balance and inner peace.

ROCK ROSE

Rock Rose is one of the 38 Bach Flower Remedies, and it is known as the Courage Flower. This remedy is for those who experience intense and overwhelming fear, terror, or panic in the face of a crisis or traumatic event. Rock Rose can help to bring calm and courage to those who feel paralyzed by fear and unable to cope with the situation at hand.

The essence of Rock Rose is extracted from the flowers of the Rock Rose plant, which grows wild in the rocky terrain of southern Europe. This beautiful yellow flower is known for its resilience and ability to thrive in harsh conditions, making it a symbol of courage and strength.

Rock Rose is particularly effective for those who are experiencing a sudden and unexpected crisis, such as an accident, natural disaster, or medical emergency. It can also be helpful for those who suffer from recurring nightmares or flashbacks related to past traumatic experiences.

When taken as a Bach Flower Remedy, Rock Rose can help to restore a sense of inner strength and calm in the face of adversity. It can help to bring clarity to the mind and allow for a more rational and practical approach to problem-solving. It can also help to reduce the physical symptoms of anxiety, such as trembling, sweating, and a racing heart.

Rock Rose is a powerful remedy that can help to restore courage and resilience in even the most difficult of circumstances. It is a reminder that even in the face of overwhelming fear, we have the inner resources to overcome our challenges and emerge stronger on the other side.

If you are experiencing intense fear or anxiety related to a crisis or traumatic event, Rock Rose may be the remedy for you. It can be taken alone or in combination with other Bach Flower Remedies to address specific emotional and mental states. It is a safe and natural remedy that can be taken by anyone, regardless of age or medical history.

In summary, Rock Rose is a powerful and effective Bach Flower Remedy that can help to restore courage and strength in the face of adversity. Its ability to bring calm and clarity to the mind can help to reduce the physical and emotional symptoms of anxiety and fear. If you are seeking a natural and holistic approach to emotional and mental wellness, consider incorporating Rock Rose into your daily routine. With the Courage Flower on your side, you can face any challenge with confidence and resilience.

Rock Water Bach Flower Remedy is a unique and powerful remedy that can help us in our journey towards emotional and physical wellness. This remedy is specifically designed for individuals who are strict and hard on themselves, often holding themselves to impossibly high standards. The remedy is meant to help these individuals release their inner rigidity, allowing them to live more freely and authentically.

The essence of Rock Water is found in the natural springs that bubble up from the earth, full of energy and vitality. This essence is then captured and distilled into a potent remedy that can help us in our own personal growth and transformation. The remedy is known to help us release our fears and anxieties, enabling us to live with more courage and confidence.

The benefits of Rock Water Bach Flower Remedy are many. It can help us overcome feelings of self-doubt and inadequacy, allowing us to be more comfortable in our own skin. It can also help us break free from self-imposed limitations, enabling us to pursue our dreams and aspirations with greater passion and purpose.

Another benefit of Rock Water is that it can help us become more adaptable and flexible. When we are too rigid and inflexible, we can become stuck in our ways and resistant to change. But with the help of Rock Water, we can learn to embrace new ideas and experiences, and move more fluidly through life's challenges.

Furthermore, Rock Water can help us become more compassionate and forgiving towards ourselves. Often, we are our own harshest critics, and we hold ourselves to standards that are impossible to meet. But with the help of this remedy, we can learn to accept ourselves as we are, flaws and all, and treat ourselves with the kindness and compassion we deserve.

In conclusion, Rock Water Bach Flower Remedy is a powerful tool for personal growth and transformation. By helping us release our inner rigidity and embrace new experiences and ideas, we can become more adaptable, compassionate, and courageous. If you are someone who is hard on yourself and struggles with feelings of self-doubt and inadequacy, I highly recommend giving this remedy a try. It has the potential to transform your life in ways you never thought possible.

SCLERANTHUS

Life is a rollercoaster ride of ups and downs, and it's not always easy to keep our balance. One moment we may feel on top of the world, and the next we may be plunged into doubt and indecision. When we find ourselves in these situations, it can be challenging to make a decision and move forward. That's where the Scleranthus Bach Flower Remedy comes in - this remedy can help us find balance in the face of life's uncertainties.

Scleranthus is a remedy that helps us overcome indecision and find our inner compass. If you're the kind of person who struggles to make decisions, whether they are big or small, Scleranthus can help you find the clarity you need to move forward. It helps to bring balance to the inner emotional state, which can be skewed due to conflicting desires or hesitancy to make a choice.

This remedy can also be useful for those who tend to fluctuate between extremes. Perhaps you find yourself vacillating between feelings of happiness and sadness or between being outgoing and introverted. If this is the case, Scleranthus can help you find a middle ground and bring balance to your emotions. It can help you become more centred and grounded, allowing you to feel more stable and at ease.

In essence, Scleranthus helps us overcome our indecision and find our inner balance. It helps us to become more attuned to our emotions and to understand what we truly want. This remedy can be especially useful in situations where we are faced with tough decisions or when we're feeling overwhelmed by conflicting emotions.

When taking the Scleranthus remedy, it's essential to trust the process and allow it to work. Remember that the remedy can help you find your inner compass, but ultimately, it's up to you to make the final decision. This remedy is not meant to make decisions for you but to help you find the clarity and balance you need to make the right choice.

In conclusion, the Scleranthus Bach Flower Remedy can help us find balance in the face of life's uncertainties. It can help us overcome indecision, become more centred, and find our inner compass. By bringing balance to our emotions, we can find a middle ground and become more stable and at ease. So if you find yourself struggling with indecision or fluctuating between extremes, consider trying Scleranthus and discover the peace and balance that it can bring to your life.

STAR OF BETHLEHEM

Star of Bethlehem, also known as Ornithogalum umbellatum, is one of the 38 remedies that make up the Bach Flower Remedies system. This remedy is designed to help those who have experienced trauma or shock, whether it be physical or emotional.

The trauma or shock that Star of Bethlehem aims to address may be recent or long-standing, and can have a profound impact on an individual's physical and emotional wellbeing. This trauma can manifest in various ways, such as anxiety, depression, insomnia, and even physical symptoms like headaches or digestive issues.

The Star of Bethlehem remedy works by helping to soothe and heal the mind and body, allowing individuals to process and release the trauma they have experienced. This can bring a sense of calm and inner peace, and can help individuals regain a sense of control over their lives.

When taking the Star of Bethlehem remedy, individuals may experience a sense of release, both physically and emotionally. This can lead to a greater sense of clarity, and may help them to move past the trauma they have experienced. They may also find that they are better able to cope with future stress and adversity, as they have developed greater resilience and emotional strength.

It is important to note that the Star of Bethlehem remedy is not a replacement for professional medical care or therapy. However, it can be a useful tool in a holistic approach to healing and self-care. By incorporating the Star of Bethlehem remedy into a broader self-care routine, individuals may find that they are better able to manage their symptoms and maintain their overall wellbeing.

Overall, the Star of Bethlehem Bach Flower Remedy is a powerful tool for those who have experienced trauma or shock. By addressing the root cause of their symptoms, individuals can experience a greater sense of peace and wellbeing, and may be better equipped to handle future challenges. Whether used alone or in combination with other remedies, Star of Bethlehem can be an invaluable tool in the journey towards healing and self-discovery.

SWEET CHESTNUT

Sweet Chestnut is a powerful Bach Flower Remedy that can bring about miraculous renewal to those who feel they have reached the end of their tether. If you feel that you have reached the absolute limits of your endurance, that there is no hope left, or that your life is so dark and bleak that there can be no way out, then Sweet Chestnut may be the answer you have been looking for.

Sweet Chestnut is often referred to as the "Bach Flower of Last Hope." It is for those moments when we have tried everything we know to do, and nothing seems to work. When we have reached the point of complete despair and hopelessness, Sweet Chestnut can come to the rescue, bringing about a profound shift in our inner landscape.

Sweet Chestnut is not a remedy for the faint-hearted. It is for those who are willing to go through the dark night of the soul, to face their deepest fears, and to emerge renewed and transformed. This remedy can help us to let go of old patterns and beliefs that no longer serve us, and to embrace a new way of being that is more aligned with our true selves.

When we take Sweet Chestnut, we may feel as though we are being stripped down to our very core. We may feel as though we are being put through a crucible, burning away all that is false and leaving only what is true. We may feel as though we are facing our darkest fears and our deepest wounds, but through it all, there is a sense of hope and renewal that shines like a beacon in the darkness.

Sweet Chestnut is a remedy for those who have been through the fire and have emerged stronger and more resilient. It is a reminder that even in our darkest moments, there is always hope. That even when we feel as though we have nothing left, there is always a wellspring of strength within us that we can draw upon.

If you are facing a difficult time in your life, if you feel as though there is no way out, then Sweet Chestnut may be the remedy you need. This Bach Flower Remedy can help you to connect with your inner strength and resilience, to let go of what no longer serves you, and to emerge renewed and transformed. So, take heart, my friend, and know that even in the darkest moments, there is always a light that shines within.

VERVAIN

Vervain is a Bach Flower Remedy that is known for its ability to help individuals who are extremely passionate, enthusiastic, and have strong convictions. Those who benefit from this remedy often feel as if they are on a mission or have a purpose in life and will stop at nothing to achieve it. This passion can be a great asset, but when it becomes excessive, it can lead to burnout and exhaustion.

People who need Vervain are often highly opinionated and can come across as preachy or dogmatic. They may have trouble listening to others and accepting different viewpoints, and may even become frustrated or angry when others do not share their level of enthusiasm or commitment. Vervain types are often highly driven and may push themselves to the point of exhaustion or illness.

The Vervain remedy can help these individuals to find a balance between their strong convictions and the needs and opinions of others. It can help to calm their intensity and help them to be more open-minded and accepting of different perspectives. Vervain can also help them to take a step back and evaluate whether their passion and enthusiasm are truly serving them and their goals or if they are causing them harm.

One of the key benefits of Vervain is its ability to help individuals find a sense of inner calm and balance. When taken regularly, Vervain can help to reduce feelings of stress, tension, and frustration, and promote a greater sense of peace and relaxation. This can be especially helpful for those who struggle with anxiety, nervousness, or insomnia.

Another benefit of Vervain is its ability to promote greater empathy and understanding towards others. As those who take Vervain become more balanced and centred, they may find it easier to listen to others and accept different viewpoints. They may also find it easier to express themselves in a calm and measured way, rather than becoming overly emotional or aggressive.

In summary, Vervain is a Bach Flower Remedy that can be a powerful tool for those who are highly passionate, enthusiastic, and driven. By helping to calm their intensity and promote greater empathy and balance, Vervain can help these individuals to achieve their goals without burning themselves out or becoming overwhelmed. If you find yourself struggling with a sense of extreme conviction or a need to always be on the go, Vervain may be the remedy you need to find greater peace, balance, and fulfilment in your life.

<u>VINE</u>

Vine Bach Flower Remedy is one of the most powerful remedies within the Bach Flower system. Its effects can be profound, offering a sense of clarity, purpose, and strength to those who use it.

The essence of Vine is all about finding inner strength and asserting oneself in a positive and productive way. It is especially useful for those who feel overwhelmed or uncertain about their place in the world, helping them to connect with their inner power and take action towards their goals.

Vine is an excellent remedy for those who struggle with authority or who have a tendency to dominate others. It can help to balance out these tendencies and promote a more collaborative, cooperative approach to leadership. At the same time, it can also help those who feel powerless or submissive to stand up for themselves and assert their needs.

One of the most remarkable things about Vine is its ability to help people tap into their creativity and inner wisdom. By promoting a sense of confidence and self-assurance, Vine can help individuals to access their innate talents and gifts, bringing them to the surface for the benefit of all.

Whether you are a student struggling to find your place in the world, an entrepreneur looking to take your business to the next level, or simply someone seeking to connect with your inner power and potential, Vine Bach Flower Remedy can help. Its effects are gentle but profound, offering a sense of clarity, focus, and purpose to those who use it.

To use Vine, simply add a few drops to a glass of water and sip throughout the day. You can also add it to a spray bottle and mist around your home or office for an added boost of energy and inspiration. Whatever method you choose, be sure to take Vine regularly and with an open mind, allowing its healing powers to work their magic in your life.

In conclusion, Vine Bach Flower Remedy is a powerful tool for anyone seeking to connect with their inner strength and purpose. Its effects are gentle but profound, helping to promote a sense of clarity, confidence, and creativity in those who use it. Whether you are struggling with authority issues or simply seeking to tap into your innate talents and gifts, Vine can help. So why not give it a try and see what wonders it can work in your life?

<u>WALNUT</u>

Change can be a challenging and unsettling experience, whether we initiate it ourselves or it comes unexpectedly. We may find ourselves facing uncertainty, fear, and doubt as we navigate the unknown territory ahead. However, change is a natural and necessary part of life, and with the right mindset and support, we can learn to embrace it as an opportunity for growth and transformation.

This is where Walnut Bach Flower Remedy comes in. Walnut is a powerful tool for those who are going through a period of transition, whether it's a new job, a move to a new place, the end of a relationship, or any other major life change. It helps us to let go of the past and adapt to new circumstances with grace and ease.

One of the key benefits of Walnut is that it strengthens our sense of self and our ability to stay true to our own path, even in the face of external pressures and influences. It helps us to break free from old habits and beliefs that no longer serve us, and to embrace new opportunities with confidence and enthusiasm.

Another way in which Walnut supports us through change is by easing the emotional and physical symptoms that can arise during times of transition. It can help to alleviate anxiety, stress, and nervous tension, as well as physical symptoms such as digestive issues and skin problems that are often linked to stress.

But perhaps the most profound gift of Walnut is its ability to help us see the bigger picture of our lives. It helps us to recognize the interconnectedness of all things and to trust in the universe's plan for us, even when we can't see the way forward. By cultivating a sense of trust and surrender, we can open ourselves up to new experiences and possibilities, and allow ourselves to be guided towards our highest potential.

In short, Walnut Bach Flower Remedy is a valuable ally for anyone who is going through a period of change and transformation. By helping us to let go of the past, stay true to ourselves, and trust in the journey ahead, it can empower us to embrace new opportunities and live our lives to the fullest. So if you're feeling stuck or unsure about what the future holds, give Walnut a try and see how it can support you on your journey of growth and evolution.

<u>*WATER VIOLET*</u>

Among the many Bach Flower Remedies available, Water Violet stands out for its remarkable ability to help individuals tap into their inner strength and find peace and tranquillity amidst the chaos of daily life.

Water Violet is particularly effective for individuals who tend to withdraw from the world and seek solitude, finding comfort and solace in their own company. These individuals are often highly self-sufficient and independent, and may appear aloof or distant to others. They may be reluctant to ask for help or support, preferring to handle their problems on their own.

Despite their independence, Water Violet individuals are not necessarily unhappy or discontented. Rather, they may simply value their privacy and solitude more than social interaction, and find solace in activities such as reading, writing, or meditation.

However, prolonged periods of solitude can sometimes lead to feelings of isolation or loneliness, and Water Violet individuals may struggle to connect with others or form meaningful relationships. This can be particularly challenging in today's fast-paced and interconnected world, where social interaction is often viewed as essential for success and happiness.

Fortunately, Water Violet Bach Flower Remedy can help to break down the barriers that prevent individuals from connecting with others and finding their place in the world. By promoting a sense of inner strength and tranquility, this remedy can help individuals to open themselves up to new experiences and opportunities, and embrace the richness and diversity of life.

Water Violet can be particularly helpful for individuals who are going through periods of change or transition, such as moving to a new city or starting a new job. It can help to ease feelings of uncertainty or anxiety, and provide a sense of stability and security in the midst of upheaval.

For those who are struggling to connect with others, Water Violet can help to promote empathy and understanding, and encourage individuals to reach out and form meaningful relationships. It can also help to alleviate feelings of loneliness or isolation, and provide a sense of comfort and support during difficult times.

In summary, Water Violet is an essential remedy for individuals who value their privacy and solitude, but may struggle to connect with others or find their place in the world. With its ability to promote inner strength and tranquillity, this remedy can help individuals to open themselves up to new experiences and opportunities, and embrace the richness and diversity of life. So, if you find yourself withdrawing from the world and seeking solace in solitude, consider trying Water Violet Bach Flower Remedy and unlock the power of your inner strength today.

WHITE CHESTNUT

Welcome to the world of White Chestnut Bach Flower Remedy, where peace of mind and mental clarity are just a few drops away. In this chapter, we will explore the benefits and uses of this amazing remedy, and discover how it can help you overcome the incessant chatter of your mind, bringing calm and serenity to your inner world.

White Chestnut is the perfect remedy for those who are plagued by unwanted thoughts, mental arguments, and repetitive worries that seem to never go away. It is an excellent choice for those who find it hard to switch off their minds, even during relaxation or sleep.

This remedy works by soothing the overactive mind, releasing the mental tension and restoring inner harmony. It helps you to regain control of your thoughts and emotions, enabling you to focus on the present moment and feel more connected to your inner self.

With White Chestnut Bach Flower Remedy, you will be able to let go of the incessant mental chatter that keeps you stuck in a cycle of worry and anxiety. You will find that you can now approach problems and challenges with a clear and focused mind, without getting distracted by negative thoughts or inner conflicts.

One of the greatest benefits of White Chestnut Bach Flower Remedy is that it can help you get a good night's sleep. By calming the mind and easing the tension, it allows you to drift off into a deep and restful slumber, free from the worries that keep you awake at night.

Whether you are facing a difficult decision, feeling overwhelmed, or simply need to clear your mind, White Chestnut Bach Flower Remedy can help you find the peace and tranquillity you seek. It is safe and gentle, and can be used by people of all ages, including children and pets.

In conclusion, White Chestnut Bach Flower Remedy is an excellent choice for anyone who struggles with unwanted thoughts, mental chatter, and repetitive worries. It is a powerful tool that can help you restore inner peace and mental clarity, allowing you to live your life to the fullest. So why wait? Try White Chestnut Bach Flower Remedy today and experience the joys of a calm and focused mind!

<u>*WILD OAT*</u>

Are you feeling lost or unsure about your life path? Do you find yourself constantly seeking new opportunities and experiences, but never quite finding the right fit? If so, you may be in need of Wild Oat Bach Flower Remedy.

Wild Oat is a powerful remedy that can help you find your true calling and achieve a sense of purpose and direction in your life. This remedy is particularly helpful for those who feel adrift or unsatisfied in their current job or life situation, and who are searching for a deeper sense of fulfilment.

The beauty of Wild Oat is that it can help you tune into your inner voice and connect with your true passions and interests. By aligning your actions and choices with your authentic self, you can create a life that is truly fulfilling and satisfying.

One of the key benefits of Wild Oat Bach Flower Remedy is its ability to provide clarity and focus. If you've been feeling overwhelmed or scattered in your thoughts and actions, Wild Oat can help you cut through the noise and hone in on what truly matters.

With Wild Oat, you can also gain a greater sense of confidence and self-assurance. By trusting in yourself and your own intuition, you can make decisions that align with your true desires and goals. This can lead to a greater sense of purpose and fulfilment in all areas of your life, from your career to your relationships.

So, if you're feeling lost or unsure about your path in life, consider giving Wild Oat Bach Flower Remedy a try. With its powerful ability to connect you with your inner self and provide clarity and focus, it may be just what you need to find your true calling and achieve a sense of purpose and direction in your life.

<u>*WILD ROSE*</u>

If you are looking for a way to restore your vitality and rediscover your passion for life, Wild Rose Bach Flower Remedy may be just what you need. This powerful remedy can help you break free from apathy and find renewed purpose and enthusiasm.

Wild Rose is a Bach Flower Remedy that is specifically designed to address a lack of interest in life. This can manifest in various ways, such as feeling bored or disinterested in daily activities, lacking motivation or drive, or feeling resigned to a dull and unfulfilling existence. If any of these symptoms resonate with you, Wild Rose could be the perfect solution.

One of the key benefits of Wild Rose Bach Flower Remedy is that it helps to reconnect us with our inner sense of purpose and passion. When we lose sight of what truly matters to us, we can become disconnected from our own sense of identity and sense of self. Wild Rose helps to reignite that spark and bring us back in touch with our deepest desires and aspirations.

Another wonderful thing about Wild Rose Bach Flower Remedy is that it works on a deep emotional level. This remedy is not simply a temporary fix, but rather a means of addressing the root cause of our lack of interest in life. By working to heal the emotional imbalances that underpin our feelings of apathy, Wild Rose can help us to achieve long-lasting and meaningful change.

Perhaps one of the most compelling things about Wild Rose Bach Flower Remedy is that it is completely natural and non-invasive. Unlike many conventional treatments, Wild Rose does not come with a host of unwanted side effects or risks. Instead, it offers a gentle and holistic approach to healing that can be integrated seamlessly into your daily routine.

Incorporating Wild Rose Bach Flower Remedy into your life is easy and convenient. Simply add a few drops to your water, or place a few drops under your tongue several times a day. You can also add it to your bath water, or use it in a diffuser to infuse your living space with its healing properties.

Wild Rose Bach Flower Remedy is a powerful and effective tool for anyone seeking to rediscover their passion for life. By working to heal the emotional imbalances that lead to apathy and disinterest, Wild Rose can help you to find renewed energy, purpose, and enthusiasm.

<u>WILLOW</u>

The Willow Bach Flower Remedy is a powerful tool for those who struggle with resentment, bitterness, and blame. If you often feel victimized by life, and find yourself frequently complaining about your circumstances, Willow can help you shift your perspective and find gratitude and forgiveness.

The key to understanding Willow's power lies in its ability to connect us with the natural ebb and flow of life. Life is not always easy, and we all face challenges and setbacks along the way. However, it's our response to these challenges that ultimately determines our level of happiness and fulfilment. If we allow ourselves to become trapped in a cycle of blame and bitterness, we create a self-fulfilling prophecy that only leads to more unhappiness and disappointment.

Willow helps us break this cycle by encouraging us to take responsibility for our own emotions and reactions. It helps us see that we are not victims of circumstance, but rather active participants in our own lives. By embracing this truth, we can begin to let go of our resentments and find gratitude for the blessings we do have.

One of the key benefits of Willow is its ability to promote forgiveness. Holding onto grudges and resentments only creates more pain and suffering in our lives. When we hold onto anger and bitterness, we are only hurting ourselves. Willow helps us release these negative emotions and find forgiveness, both for ourselves and for others. This can be a powerful tool for healing old wounds and restoring relationships that may have been damaged by past hurts.

Another benefit of Willow is its ability to help us find perspective. When we are caught up in the midst of our own struggles and challenges, it can be difficult to see the bigger picture. Willow helps us step back and see our situation with fresh eyes. This can help us find new solutions and approaches to our problems, and can also help us appreciate the blessings we do have in our lives.

If you are struggling with resentment, bitterness, or blame, Willow may be just the remedy you need. By helping you find forgiveness, gratitude, and perspective, it can help you break free from old patterns of negativity and create a brighter, more fulfilling future. So why not give it a try? With the help of Willow, you can unlock the power of forgiveness and gratitude and create a happier, more peaceful life for yourself.

Are you someone who struggles with overwhelming emotions during stressful situations? Do you find it difficult to calm your nerves and regain your composure during moments of panic or distress? If so, then Rescue Bach Flower Remedy might just be the solution you're looking for!

Rescue Remedy is a unique combination of five Bach Flower Remedies that work together to help soothe and calm the mind and body. These five remedies - Rock Rose, Impatiens, Cherry Plum, Star of Bethlehem, and Clematis - each address different aspects of emotional distress, such as fear, impatience, or shock.

The Rock Rose flower, for example, is known for its ability to alleviate extreme fear and panic, while Impatiens helps to ease impatience and irritability. Cherry Plum addresses feelings of loss of control, while Star of Bethlehem is particularly effective in dealing with the shock of a traumatic event. Finally, Clematis can help to bring focus and clarity to the mind, particularly in situations where one may feel detached or ungrounded.

The beauty of Rescue Remedy is its versatility - it can be used in a variety of situations where emotional stress is a factor. Whether you're facing an exam or job interview, experiencing grief or trauma, or dealing with anxiety or panic attacks, Rescue Remedy can provide a sense of calm and comfort.

One of the best things about Rescue Remedy is its ease of use. Whether in the form of drops, spray, or pastilles, it can be taken directly or added to water or other beverages. It can also be applied topically, such as on the temples or wrists, for more immediate relief.

So if you're looking for a natural and effective way to cope with stress and emotional distress, Rescue Remedy may be just the thing for you. With its unique combination of Bach Flower Remedies, it can provide relief from a variety of negative emotions and bring a sense of calm and balance to your life.

In conclusion, Rescue Remedy is a powerful tool for anyone looking to manage their emotional well-being. Its combination of Bach Flower Remedies can provide relief from a variety of negative emotions, and its ease of use makes it a convenient and accessible solution. So why not give it a try and discover the healing powers of Rescue Remedy for yourself?

"Important note regarding all the Bach Flower Remedy Chapters: Each chapter is self-contained, allowing you the flexibility to read them in any order that suits you. As a Portuguese speaker, I have received assistance from my friends and software to write in English. This may lead to instances where you feel that the same information is being repeated intentionally."

As the sun rises on a new day, we are faced with countless choices. What to wear, what to eat, and how to spend our time are just a few examples of the many decisions we make every day. However, some choices are more important than others, and choosing the right remedy to address your emotional needs is one of them.

When it comes to choosing the right remedy from the Bach Flower Remedies system, there are several factors to consider. First and foremost, it's essential to understand your emotional state and the specific issue you're looking to address. Each remedy is designed to help with a specific emotional state, so it's crucial to choose the remedy that aligns with your emotional needs.

Another critical factor to consider is the intensity of your emotions. If you're experiencing strong, overwhelming emotions, you may need a more potent remedy to help balance and restore emotional harmony. Conversely, if your emotions are milder or fleeting, a gentler remedy may be more appropriate.

It's also important to consider the duration of your emotional state. If you've been experiencing the same emotional state for an extended period, a more long-term approach may be necessary. Alternatively, if your emotions are more temporary, a short-term remedy may be sufficient.

When selecting a remedy, it's essential to trust your intuition and listen to your body. Pay attention to any physical sensations or emotional responses you may have when considering a particular remedy. Your body may be sending you signals that can guide you towards the remedy that will be most effective for you.

Finally, it's worth noting that selecting a remedy is not a one-time event. As we continue to evolve and grow, our emotional needs and states may change. It's essential to re-evaluate our emotional states regularly and choose the appropriate remedies accordingly.

In conclusion, choosing the right Bach Flower Remedy is a deeply personal and intuitive process that requires careful consideration of several factors. By understanding your emotional needs, the intensity and duration of your emotional state, and listening to your body's signals, you can select the remedy that will best support your emotional healing and wellbeing.

While Bach Flower Remedies can be a helpful tool in promoting emotional healing and wellbeing, it's important to note that they are not a substitute for professional therapy. While remedies can provide support and help to manage emotional states, they may not address the root causes of emotional issues.

A therapist can provide guidance and support in exploring the underlying emotional issues and help to develop strategies for long-term emotional healing. Working with a therapist can also help to identify patterns of behaviour or thought that may be contributing to emotional distress and provide tools for addressing them.

Additionally, a therapist can help to ensure that the remedies you choose are appropriate for your individual needs and that they are being used in conjunction with other treatments or medications safely.

It's important to approach emotional healing from a holistic perspective, which includes both emotional and physical aspects. While Bach Flower Remedies can be an essential tool in promoting emotional wellbeing, working with a therapist can provide additional support and guidance in achieving long-term emotional healing and overall wellbeing.

Agrimony: For those who hide their emotional pain behind a cheerful exterior.

Aspen: For those who experience vague, unexplainable fears and anxiety.

Beech: For those who are critical or intolerant of others.

Centaury: For those who have difficulty saying "no" and struggle to assert themselves.

Cerato: For those who lack confidence in their own judgment and rely on the opinions of others.

Cherry Plum: For those who fear losing control of their emotions or actions.

Chestnut Bud: For those who repeat the same mistakes and struggle to learn from their experiences.

Chicory: For those who are overly possessive or controlling of others.

Clematis: For those who have a tendency to daydream or live in their own world.

Crab Apple: For those who feel unclean or ashamed and struggle with self-acceptance.

Elm: For those who feel overwhelmed or burdened by responsibility.

Gentian: For those who become easily discouraged or disheartened by setbacks.

Gorse: For those who feel hopeless and have given up on finding a solution to their problems.

Heather: For those who are overly talkative or attention-seeking.

Holly: For those who experience jealousy, envy, or suspicion towards others.

Honeysuckle: For those who dwell on the past and struggle to move on.

Hornbeam: For those who feel tired or exhausted but struggle to get started on tasks.

Impatiens: For those who are impatient or easily frustrated.

Larch: For those who lack confidence in their own abilities.

Mimulus: For those who experience specific fears or phobias.

Mustard: For those who experience deep sadness or depression without any apparent cause.

Oak: For those who persist through difficulty and become exhausted or burnt out.

Olive: For those who feel drained or exhausted and struggle to regain energy.

Pine: For those who feel guilty or responsible for things that are outside of their control.

Red Chestnut: For those who experience excessive worry or fear for the safety of others.

Rock Rose: For those who experience intense fear or terror.

Rock Water: For those who are rigid in their beliefs or lifestyle.

Scleranthus: For those who struggle to make decisions or are indecisive.

Star of Bethlehem: For those who have experienced shock or trauma.

Sweet Chestnut: For those who experience extreme emotional pain or anguish.

Vervain: For those who are overly enthusiastic or passionate and struggle to relax.

Vine: For those who are domineering or controlling towards others.

Walnut: For those who are going through a period of transition or change.

Water Violet: For those who are independent or reserved and struggle to connect with others.

White Chestnut: For those who experience persistent or unwanted thoughts.

Wild Oat: For those who struggle to find direction or purpose in life.

Wild Rose: For those who feel apathetic or resigned to their circumstances.

Willow: For those who feel resentful or bitter towards others or life circumstances.

To sum up, selecting the appropriate Bach Flower Remedy requires a thorough understanding of the emotional states each remedy is designed to address. By choosing the remedy that aligns with our emotional needs, we can promote emotional healing and overall wellbeing. For a more detailed understanding of each Bach Flower Remedy, I recommend revisiting each remedy's chapter.

THE HEALING PROCESS

Emotional healing and wellbeing are essential aspects of a happy and fulfilling life. Unfortunately, navigating the ups and downs of life can be challenging, and many of us struggle with emotional issues at some point in our lives. Whether you're struggling with anxiety, depression, grief, or any other emotional issue, the journey towards emotional healing and wellbeing can be a transformative and empowering experience.

Bach Flower Remedies offer a unique and natural approach to promoting emotional healing and wellbeing. The remedies work by addressing specific emotional states, promoting emotional balance, and restoring harmony to the mind and body. They are gentle, safe, and can be used in conjunction with other treatments or medications.

The beauty of Bach Flower Remedies is that they are designed to support the unique emotional needs of each individual. By understanding the emotional states each remedy addresses, we can select the remedies that best align with our emotional needs and support our overall wellbeing.

The healing journey with Bach Flower Remedies is a unique and deeply personal experience. It requires self-awareness, self-care, and a willingness to explore and reflect on our emotional states and triggers. The journey towards emotional healing can be challenging, but it can also be a transformative and empowering experience.

One of the most critical aspects of the healing journey involves developing a heightened sense of self-awareness. By gaining a deeper understanding of our emotional states and triggers, we can gain valuable insights into our needs and select the most appropriate remedies to facilitate our emotional healing. This process may involve delving into past experiences, analysing behavioural or thought patterns, and engaging in mindful self-reflection.

Another fundamental component of the healing journey is self-nurturance. Self-care can take various forms, such as maintaining adequate sleep, following a nutritious diet, engaging in routine physical activity, and taking regular breaks to relax and re-energize. Prioritizing self-nurturance is crucial to sustaining our overall well-being and making it a habit in our everyday lives.

Seeking the assistance of a therapist can also be a valuable asset in the healing process. By collaborating with a therapist, we can access guidance and support in exploring our emotional issues, honing our coping mechanisms, and cultivating long-lasting emotional wellness.

It is critical to approach the healing journey with a receptive mindset and an open heart. While the journey towards emotional healing may be arduous, it can ultimately lead to a profound transformation and a sense of empowerment. By keeping an open mind and exposing ourselves to new experiences and perspectives, we can foster resilience, growth, and emotional prosperity.

Therefore, Bach Flower Remedies offer an exceptional and natural approach to supporting emotional healing and overall

<u>Developing a Holistic Approach to Wellness with Bach Flower Remedies</u>

In today's world, the concept of wellness has expanded beyond mere physical health. Holistic wellness encompasses multiple dimensions, including emotional, social, intellectual, spiritual, and occupational wellness. Bach Flower Remedies offer a unique and natural approach to holistic wellness, targeting the emotional dimension to facilitate emotional healing and promote overall well-being.

To develop a holistic approach to wellness with Bach Flower Remedies, it's essential to understand the interconnectedness of various dimensions of wellness. Emotional health is closely linked to physical, social, and spiritual wellness. Negative emotional states can manifest themselves physically, leading to symptoms such as headaches, digestive issues, or muscle tension. Conversely, unhealthy physical states can result in emotional issues such as anxiety, stress, or depression.

The use of Bach Flower Remedies can help address emotional issues and promote holistic wellness. Bach Flower Remedies facilitate the release of negative emotions, allowing individuals to feel more at peace and better able to manage their emotions. By promoting emotional healing, Bach Flower Remedies can help individuals break the negative cycle between emotional and physical health.

To develop a holistic approach to wellness with Bach Flower Remedies, it's essential to incorporate various self-care practices into our daily routine. Regular exercise, healthy eating habits, stress-management techniques, and prioritizing emotional self-care are examples of self-care practices that can promote holistic wellness.

Emotional self-care practices can include mindfulness, meditation, journaling, or engaging in activities that promote positive emotions, such as spending time in nature, practicing gratitude, or engaging in hobbies or creative pursuits.

Working with a Bach Flower Remedies therapist can also be a valuable component of a holistic approach to wellness. A therapist can help identify the appropriate remedies for an individual's emotional needs, support emotional healing, and offer guidance on developing healthy self-care practices. A therapist can also provide support and encouragement, helping individuals stay on track with their self-care and emotional healing journey.

Bach Flower Remedies offer a unique and natural approach to promoting holistic wellness by targeting the emotional dimension. To develop a holistic approach to wellness with Bach Flower Remedies, it's essential to understand the interconnectedness of various dimensions of wellness and prioritize self-care practices. By incorporating Bach Flower Remedies into our self-care routine and seeking guidance from a therapist, we can promote emotional healing, achieve balance, and attain overall well-being. A holistic approach to wellness with Bach Flower Remedies can be transformative, empowering, and life-changing. I invite you to join me on this journey towards holistic wellness and emotional healing with Bach Flower Remedies.

As we go through life, we encounter a variety of stressors that can impact our emotional and physical health. These stressors can range from daily pressures and challenges to major life changes, trauma, and illness. To support our overall wellbeing, it's essential to practice self-care and develop a holistic approach to wellness, including managing emotional and physical detox.

Detoxification is the process of removing toxins and other harmful substances from the body. Emotional and physical detox involve releasing negative emotions, thoughts, and behaviours that no longer serve us and replacing them with positive and empowering ones. Bach Flower Remedies can be a powerful tool to support emotional and physical detoxification.

To manage emotional detox, it's essential to identify and acknowledge the negative emotions that we may be holding onto, such as fear, anger, resentment, and sadness. Once we identify these emotions, we can select the appropriate Bach Flower Remedies to support our emotional healing. For example, if we're experiencing fear and anxiety, we may benefit from using Mimulus or Aspen. If we're feeling overwhelmed and stressed, we may benefit from using Rescue Remedy. By using Bach Flower Remedies to address our emotional needs, we can support the process of emotional detoxification.

Physical detox involves eliminating toxins and harmful substances from our bodies. This can be achieved through a variety of practices, such as eating a healthy diet, exercising regularly, staying hydrated, and reducing exposure to environmental toxins. Bach Flower Remedies can also support physical detox by addressing the emotional and mental factors that contribute to physical illness and disease. For example, if we're experiencing chronic stress, we may benefit from using Agrimony or Vervain to support relaxation and reduce tension.

It's important to approach emotional and physical detox with patience and self-compassion. The process of detoxification can be challenging, and it's essential to give ourselves the time and space to heal. We can support our detoxification process by practicing self-care, such as getting enough sleep, eating a healthy diet, and engaging in regular physical activity.

Managing emotional and physical detox is a crucial part of developing a holistic approach to wellness. Bach Flower Remedies can be a powerful tool to support emotional and physical detoxification. By identifying and acknowledging negative emotions and using the appropriate Bach Flower Remedies, we can support our emotional healing. By practicing self-care and reducing exposure to environmental toxins, we can support our physical detoxification. I invite you to explore the benefits of Bach Flower Remedies and develop a holistic approach to emotional and physical wellness.

Below are a few examples that demonstrate the practical application of Bach Remedies.

anxiety and depression

One of the most commonly used Bach Flower Remedies for anxiety and depression is Rescue Remedy. This remedy is a combination of five different Bach Flower Remedies, including Impatiens, Star of Bethlehem, Cherry Plum, Rock Rose, and Clematis. It's designed to help manage feelings of panic, fear, and overwhelm, making it an excellent option for those experiencing anxiety or depression.

Another Bach Flower Remedy that can be helpful for anxiety and depression is White Chestnut. This remedy is designed to help quiet the mind and alleviate persistent or racing thoughts that can contribute to feelings of anxiety and depression. It's an excellent option for those who struggle with racing thoughts or find it challenging to quiet their mind.

Mimulus is another Bach Flower Remedy that can be helpful for anxiety. This remedy is designed to help manage fear and anxiety related to specific situations or phobias, making it an excellent option for those who experience anxiety related to specific triggers or situations.

For those struggling with depression, Gentian can be an excellent option. This remedy is designed to help manage feelings of discouragement or hopelessness and can be helpful for those who struggle with negative thinking patterns or low self-esteem.

Additionally, Mustard can be a helpful remedy for those experiencing depression. This remedy is designed to help manage feelings of sadness or depression that come and go without an apparent cause. It can be helpful for those who experience depressive episodes that seem to come out of nowhere.

It's important to note that Bach Flower Remedies are not a substitute for professional medical treatment, and those experiencing severe anxiety or depression should seek the help of a healthcare professional. However, for those experiencing mild to moderate symptoms, Bach Flower Remedies can be a safe and effective way to manage symptoms naturally and holistically.

When using Bach Flower Remedies for anxiety or depression, it's essential to choose the remedies that best align with your specific symptoms and emotional needs. Working with a Bach Flower Remedy practitioner or knowledgeable healthcare professional can help ensure that you're choosing the right remedies and using them correctly.

Bach Flower Remedies can be a safe and effective way to manage symptoms of anxiety and depression naturally and holistically. By choosing the remedies that best align with your specific symptoms and emotional needs, you can support your overall emotional wellbeing and promote a sense of calm and balance in your life.

grief and loss

The experience of grief and loss is an inevitable part of life, and everyone goes through it at some point. Whether it's the loss of a loved one, a job, a relationship, or even a pet, the emotional pain and stress can be overwhelming. It's essential to understand that everyone's grieving process is unique, and there is no right or wrong way to grieve. However, Bach Flower Remedies can provide support and ease the emotional pain during this difficult time.

The Bach Flower Remedy most commonly used for grief and loss is Star of Bethlehem. This remedy is particularly helpful in easing the shock and trauma that often accompanies sudden loss or unexpected news. Star of Bethlehem helps to restore a sense of inner peace and comfort, allowing the individual to process their emotions more effectively.

Another remedy commonly used for grief is Sweet Chestnut. This remedy is particularly useful for individuals experiencing deep and intense emotional pain, feelings of hopelessness, and a sense of despair. Sweet Chestnut can help to ease the emotional pain and promote a sense of comfort and hopefulness.

Gorse is another Bach Flower Remedy that can be useful during times of grief and loss. This remedy is particularly helpful for individuals who are experiencing a sense of hopelessness and despair, and who feel that there is no hope for the future. Gorse can help to restore a sense of optimism and positivity, allowing the individual to move forward and find hope in the future.

Other Bach Flower Remedies that can be helpful for grief and loss include Cherry Plum, which can help to ease the fear and anxiety that often accompanies loss, and Honeysuckle, which can help individuals to let go of the past and move forward with their lives.

It's important to remember that Bach Flower Remedies are not a substitute for professional medical or therapeutic support. Still, they can provide support and ease the emotional pain during difficult times. If you're struggling with grief and loss, it's essential to seek out the support of a licensed therapist or counsellor who can provide guidance and support as you navigate your emotions.

Bach Flower Remedies can provide support and ease the emotional pain during times of grief and loss. The remedies can help to restore a sense of inner peace and comfort, promote a sense of optimism and positivity, and allow individuals to move forward and find hope in the future. If you're struggling with grief and loss, I encourage you to explore the use of Bach Flower Remedies as part of your overall emotional support and healing journey.

stress and burnout

In today's fast-paced world, stress and burnout have become common problems for many people. From work pressure to family responsibilities, the demands of modern life can leave us feeling overwhelmed and exhausted. Fortunately, Bach Remedies offer a natural and effective solution for managing stress and preventing burnout.

Stress is a natural response to challenging situations, and it can motivate us to take action and solve problems. However, chronic stress can lead to physical and emotional exhaustion, and if left unchecked, it can contribute to burnout. Burnout is a state of emotional, physical, and mental exhaustion that results from prolonged stress.

Bach Remedies can help manage stress and prevent burnout by addressing the emotional root causes of these conditions. Each remedy is designed to address a specific emotional state, such as fear, anxiety, or overwhelm, that can contribute to stress and burnout.

One of the most commonly used Bach Remedies for stress and burnout is Rescue Remedy. This remedy is a combination of five different Bach Remedies and is designed to provide immediate relief from stress and anxiety. It can be taken as needed throughout the day to help manage stress and prevent burnout.

Other Bach Remedies that can be helpful for managing stress and preventing burnout include:

Elm: for overwhelm and feeling unable to cope with demands and responsibilities.
Oak: for those who work tirelessly and neglect their own self-care, leading to burnout.
White Chestnut: for racing thoughts and mental chatter that contribute to stress and prevent restful sleep.
Impatiens: for impatience and irritability, which can contribute to stress and strain relationships.
When using Bach Remedies for stress and burnout, it's important to choose remedies that address the specific emotional states that are contributing to these conditions. It's also essential to follow the recommended dosage and frequency of use for each remedy.

In addition to using Bach Remedies, it's important to practice self-care and stress management techniques to prevent burnout. This can include activities such as regular exercise, mindfulness meditation, and getting enough sleep. Seeking support from a therapist or mental health professional can also be helpful in managing stress and preventing burnout.

Bach Remedies offer a natural and effective solution for managing stress and preventing burnout. By addressing the emotional root causes of these conditions, Bach Remedies can provide relief and promote overall wellbeing. When using Bach Remedies for stress and burnout, it's important to choose remedies that address specific emotional states and to practice self-care and stress management techniques.

Using Bach Remedies for Sleep and Relaxation

Getting enough quality sleep and taking time to relax are essential for maintaining physical and emotional wellbeing. However, many people struggle with sleep-related issues, such as insomnia, sleep apnea, or restless sleep. Additionally, it can be challenging to find time to relax and unwind amidst the demands of daily life. Bach Flower Remedies can be a natural and effective way to support restful sleep and promote relaxation.

The following are some of the most commonly used Bach Remedies for sleep and relaxation:

White Chestnut - This remedy is beneficial for calming the mind and promoting peaceful thoughts, which can be especially helpful for individuals who experience racing thoughts or persistent mental chatter at bedtime.

Rescue Remedy - This combination remedy is often used for acute stress or anxiety, which can interfere with sleep. It contains a blend of five different Bach Remedies, including

Cherry Plum, Clematis, Impatiens, Rock Rose, and Star of Bethlehem.

Agrimony - This remedy can be helpful for individuals who use humor or a positive attitude to mask underlying stress or anxiety, which can interfere with restful sleep.

Aspen - This remedy is beneficial for individuals who experience vague or unknown fears that can disrupt sleep, such as nightmares or night terrors.

Vervain - This remedy can be helpful for individuals who experience physical tension and restlessness that can interfere with sleep.

To use Bach Remedies for sleep and relaxation, start by selecting the appropriate remedy or combination of remedies based on your specific symptoms or emotional state. Add two drops of the selected remedy to a glass of water and sip it slowly throughout the day or before bedtime. Alternatively, add two drops of the selected remedy to a spray bottle filled with water and mist your pillow or bedding before sleep.

It's important to note that Bach Remedies are not intended to replace medical treatment for sleep-related issues. If you are experiencing chronic or severe sleep disturbances, it's essential to speak with your healthcare provider to rule out any underlying medical conditions or to discuss treatment options.

In addition to Bach Remedies, there are several lifestyle changes that can support restful sleep and relaxation. These include:

Establishing a consistent sleep routine, including going to bed and waking up at the same time each day.

Creating a relaxing bedtime routine, such as taking a warm bath or practicing gentle yoga or stretching.

Avoiding stimulating activities before bed, such as screen time or vigorous exercise.

Creating a comfortable sleep environment, including a cool and dark bedroom, comfortable bedding, and a supportive mattress.

Practicing stress-reducing techniques, such as mindfulness meditation, deep breathing exercises, or gentle yoga.

Bach Flower Remedies can be a natural and effective way to support restful sleep and promote relaxation. By selecting the appropriate remedies based on your specific symptoms or emotional state and incorporating lifestyle changes that support sleep and relaxation, you can enhance your overall wellbeing and enjoy a more restful and rejuvenating sleep.

Bach Flower Remedies offer a unique and natural approach to emotional healing and wellbeing. One of the many benefits of these remedies is the ability to create custom blends to address specific emotional needs. By combining different Bach Flower Remedies, we can tailor our approach to emotional healing and support our overall wellbeing.

To create a custom blend, it's essential to first identify the specific emotional issues or needs that we want to address. This can involve reflecting on our emotional state, examining patterns of behaviour or thought, and considering any past traumas or experiences that may be contributing to our current emotional state.

Once we have identified our emotional needs, we can begin selecting the appropriate Bach Flower Remedies to include in our custom blend. Each Bach Flower Remedy is designed to address specific emotional states, and by selecting the appropriate remedies, we can target the emotional issues that we want to address.

For example, if we are experiencing feelings of overwhelm and anxiety, we may want to consider including remedies such as Rock Rose, Mimulus, and White Chestnut in our custom blend. Alternatively, if we are experiencing feelings of sadness and grief, we may want to include remedies such as Star of Bethlehem, Willow, and Sweet Chestnut.

When creating a custom blend, it's essential to keep in mind that each remedy has a unique role to play in addressing emotional issues. It's important to select remedies that complement each other and work together to support emotional healing.

To use the custom blend, take four drops four times a day or as needed. The drops can be taken directly under the tongue or added to a glass of water. It's essential to shake the bottle well before each use to ensure that the remedies are well mixed.

Creating a custom blend is a unique and personal approach to emotional healing with Bach Flower Remedies. By tailoring our approach to emotional healing, we can address specific emotional needs and support our overall wellbeing. I encourage you to explore the many possibilities of creating custom blends with Bach Flower Remedies and to discover the transformative power of these remedies for yourself.

Using Bach Flower Remedies as a Family

As social creatures, we rely heavily on our family for support, guidance, and love. But even the most loving and supportive families can face challenges that test their bonds. Whether it's a child struggling with anxiety or a parent coping with the loss of a loved one, emotional distress can take a toll on everyone involved.

That's where Bach Flower Remedies can help. With their gentle and natural approach to emotional healing, they can provide support and relief for the whole family. Here are some tips on how to use Bach Remedies as a family:

Identify the Emotions: The first step in using Bach Remedies as a family is to identify the emotions that each member is experiencing. Are there any recurring patterns of negative emotions, such as anxiety or anger? Are there specific situations that trigger emotional distress, such as going to school or work? By identifying these emotions, you can choose the appropriate Bach Remedies to address them.

Create a Personalized Plan: Once you've identified the emotions that need to be addressed, you can create a personalized plan for each family member. This might involve taking specific Bach Remedies, either individually or in combination, depending on the emotional state. It's important to note that Bach Remedies are safe and non-invasive, and can be taken alongside other forms of medication or therapy.

<u>Integrate Bach Remedies into Daily Routine</u>: To ensure consistency and effectiveness, it's important to integrate Bach Remedies into your family's daily routine. This might involve taking remedies at specific times of day, such as before bed or in the morning. It might also involve using remedies in specific situations, such as before a stressful event or during a difficult conversation.

<u>Monitor Progress</u>: As with any form of therapy, it's important to monitor progress and adjust the plan as needed. This might involve keeping a journal or diary of emotions and remedies used, and assessing the effectiveness over time. It's also important to communicate openly with each family member and adjust the plan as needed.

Bach Flower Remedies can be a valuable tool for families looking to manage their emotional well-being. By identifying emotions, creating personalized plans, integrating remedies into daily routines, and monitoring progress, families can work together to address emotional distress and bring a sense of calm and balance to their lives. So why not give it a try and see how Bach Remedies can benefit your family?

Using Bach Remedies in Animal Care

Bach Flower Remedies are not only useful for humans but also for animals. In fact, Bach Remedies can be a natural and effective way to promote emotional and physical healing in our animal companions. They work well in combination with traditional veterinary care and can be used to support our animals' emotional wellbeing.

The philosophy behind Bach Remedies is that emotional imbalances can lead to physical ailments in animals, just as they do in humans. For example, if an animal experiences fear, it can cause physical symptoms such as a racing heart, trembling, or digestive upset. By addressing the emotional imbalance with a Bach Remedy, the physical symptoms can also be alleviated.

The first step in using Bach Remedies for animals is to observe their behaviour and emotional state. Just like with humans, Bach Remedies are chosen based on the animal's emotional state rather than the physical symptoms they are experiencing. For example, if an animal is displaying signs of fear, a Remedy such as Mimulus may be appropriate. If an animal is feeling overwhelmed and stressed, a Remedy such as Rock Rose or Rescue Remedy may be helpful.

It's important to note that Bach Remedies are safe for animals and have no known side effects. They can be administered directly to the animal or added to their food or water. It's best to start with a small dose and observe the animal's response before increasing the dosage.

Bach Remedies can be used for a variety of animal conditions such as separation anxiety, fear of loud noises, aggressive behaviour, grief and loss, and more. For example, if an animal is experiencing separation anxiety, a combination of Rock Rose, Mimulus, and Honeysuckle may be helpful.

It's important to remember that Bach Remedies should not replace traditional veterinary care. They can be used in combination with veterinary treatment to promote emotional and physical healing in our animal companions. It's always best to consult with a veterinarian before using Bach Remedies for any animal condition.

Bach Remedies can be a natural and effective way to promote emotional and physical healing in our animal companions. They work by addressing the emotional imbalances that can lead to physical symptoms in animals. By observing an animal's behaviour and emotional state, we can choose the appropriate Bach Remedy to support their emotional wellbeing. As with any natural remedy, it's important to use Bach Remedies in conjunction with traditional veterinary care.

The environment we live in plays a crucial role in our physical and emotional well-being. Unfortunately, our modern world is full of environmental stressors that can take a toll on our health. From pollution to electromagnetic radiation, it's important to find ways to protect ourselves and promote environmental healing. That's where Bach Flower Remedies can help. Here are some tips on using Bach Remedies in environmental healing:

Identify the Environmental Stressors: The first step in using Bach Remedies for environmental healing is to identify the stressors that are affecting your environment. This might include pollution, noise, electromagnetic radiation, or other forms of environmental toxicity.

Choose the Appropriate Bach Remedies: Once you've identified the environmental stressors, you can choose the appropriate Bach Remedies to address them. For example, if pollution is a problem, you might consider using Crab Apple, which is known for its cleansing and purifying properties. If noise is a problem, you might consider using Impatiens, which promotes calm and patience.

Use Bach Remedies in Various Forms: Bach Remedies can be used in a variety of forms, depending on the environmental stressors. They can be used in sprays, drops, or creams to help purify the air or environment. You can also use Bach Remedies in combination with other environmental healing practices, such as aromatherapy, meditation, or feng shui.

Regular Use: Consistency is key when using Bach Remedies for environmental healing. It's important to use them regularly and incorporate them into your daily routine. By doing so, you'll be able to maintain a healthy and balanced environment.

Educate Yourself: In addition to using Bach Remedies, it's important to educate yourself on environmental healing practices. This might include learning about organic gardening, natural cleaning products, or reducing your carbon footprint. By making informed choices, you'll be able to create a healthy and sustainable environment for yourself and those around you.

Bach Flower Remedies can be a powerful tool in promoting environmental healing. By identifying environmental stressors, choosing the appropriate Bach Remedies, using them in various forms, regular use, and educating yourself, you can create a healthy and sustainable environment.

While Bach Flower Remedies can be used safely by anyone, it can be helpful to work with a trained practitioner to get the most out of your remedy selection and ensure the best possible results. A practitioner can provide guidance on the most effective remedies for your specific needs, help you navigate any potential side effects or interactions, and offer ongoing support throughout your healing journey.

Here are some tips for finding a Bach Remedies practitioner:

Check the official Bach Centre website: The Bach Centre maintains a list of registered practitioners worldwide. You can search by location or name to find a practitioner near you.

Ask for recommendations: If you know someone who has used Bach Remedies successfully, ask them for a recommendation. You can also ask alternative healthcare practitioners, such as naturopaths or acupuncturists, for their recommendations.

Research qualifications and training: Look for a practitioner who has completed a certified training program in Bach Remedies. This ensures that they have received proper education and training in the use of Bach Flower Remedies.

Consider the practitioner's approach: Different practitioners may have different approaches to working with Bach Remedies. Some may focus more on emotional issues, while others may *incorporate other healing modalities. Consider what approach feels most aligned with your needs and preferences.*

Schedule a consultation: Once you have identified a potential practitioner, schedule a consultation to discuss your needs and goals. This can help you get a sense of whether the practitioner is a good fit for you and can offer the support and guidance you need.

Working with a Bach Remedies practitioner can be a valuable part of your healing journey. Whether you are seeking support for a specific issue or looking to promote overall emotional wellbeing, a trained practitioner can help you navigate the world of Bach Flower Remedies and find the remedies that will best support your unique needs.

Frequently Asked Questions About Bach Flower Remedies

As with any natural remedy, there are often many questions and misconceptions surrounding the use of Bach Flower Remedies. Here are some of the most frequently asked questions to help clarify any doubts or concerns.

1. Are Bach Flower Remedies safe?
Yes, Bach Flower Remedies are completely safe and natural. They are made from flower essences and have no known side effects or interactions with other medications or treatments. However, it's essential to note that Bach Flower Remedies should not be used as a substitute for medical treatment or therapy.

2. How long does it take for Bach Flower Remedies to work?
The time it takes for Bach Flower Remedies to work varies depending on the individual and their emotional state. Some people may feel immediate relief, while others may take a few days or even weeks to notice a difference. Consistency is key when using Bach Flower Remedies, and it's essential to continue using them regularly for best results.

3. Can Bach Flower Remedies be used for children and pets?

Yes, Bach Flower Remedies are safe for use in children and pets. In fact, they can be especially effective in helping children and animals deal with emotional issues and stress. However, it's important to consult with a healthcare provider or veterinarian before giving Bach Flower Remedies to a child or pet.

4. *Can Bach Flower Remedies be used during pregnancy or while breastfeeding?*

Yes, Bach Flower Remedies are safe for use during pregnancy and while breastfeeding. However, it's essential to consult with a healthcare provider before using them to ensure that they are safe for both the mother and baby.

5. *How do I choose the right Bach Flower Remedy?*

Choosing the right Bach Flower Remedy involves identifying the emotional state or issue that needs to be addressed. Refer back to the Bach Flower Remedy chapter for more information on the specific emotional states each remedy addresses. You can also consult with a Bach Flower Practitioner for personalized guidance.

6. *Can I use multiple Bach Flower Remedies at once?*

Yes, it is possible to use multiple Bach Flower Remedies at once. However, it's essential to be mindful of how the remedies interact with each other and to use them in combination only under the guidance of a Bach Flower Practitioner.

7. *Can Bach Flower Remedies be used alongside other medications or treatments?*

Yes, Bach Flower Remedies can be used alongside other medications or treatments. However, it's essential to consult with a healthcare provider before using them in combination to ensure that there are no potential interactions or adverse effects.

Bach Flower Remedies are a safe and natural way to support emotional healing and wellbeing. By using them in combination with self-awareness, self-care, and therapy, we can cultivate resilience, growth, and emotional balance. If you have any further questions or concerns, consult with a healthcare provider or Bach Flower Practitioner for personalized guidance.

<u>Some Thoughts</u>

My brother used to have a wonderful orchid garden in the back of my house. In the mornings and sometimes in the late afternoons, I would go there and feel surrounded by the gentle rustling of leaves and the sweet fragrance of flowers. It was impossible not to marvel at the wonders of nature. This same nature has gifted us with herbs and flowers that possess incredible healing power. They provide a natural and gentle way to heal our emotions and soothe our souls.

Having already delved into the history, uses, and benefits of each of the Bach Flower Remedies, I now wish to share with you how you can inspire yourself with these remedies to lead a more fulfilling and joyful life.

The beauty of the Bach Flower Remedies lies in their ability to connect us with our inner selves, to help us recognize and release negative emotions, and to bring us back into balance. As we go about our daily lives, it is easy to get caught up in the hustle and bustle of the world, to become disconnected from our true selves and our deeper emotions. The Bach Flower Remedies offer us a way to reconnect with our innermost being and to find our way back to a place of peace and harmony.

To inspire yourself with Bach Flower Remedies, it is important to approach them with an open mind and a willingness to explore your emotions. Take the time to reflect on your feelings, to identify any negative emotions that may be holding you back, and to consider which remedies might be best suited to help you overcome these emotions.

Perhaps you find yourself struggling with fear and uncertainty, unable to move forward in life. In this case, the Bach Flower Remedy Mimulus might be just what you need to restore your confidence and courage.

Or maybe you are feeling overwhelmed and stressed, unable to cope with the demands of daily life. The Bach Flower Remedy Rescue Remedy can offer you a sense of calm and balance, helping you to navigate life's challenges with greater ease.

The key is to approach the Bach Flower Remedies with a sense of curiosity and wonder, to explore their unique qualities and to discover how they can help you on your personal journey.

As you begin to incorporate Bach Flower Remedies into your daily life, you may find yourself feeling more centred, more at ease, and more in tune with your emotions. You may discover new aspects of yourself, new strengths and insights that you had never before recognized.

In this way, the Bach Flower Remedies can serve as a powerful tool for personal growth and transformation, helping you to lead a more fulfilling and joyful life.

So go ahead, embrace the wonder and beauty of the Bach Flower Remedies, and let them inspire you to new heights of emotional wellbeing and personal fulfilment.

<u>*Piece of Advice*</u>

I want to share with you a valuable piece of advice, one that has the potential to change your life forever. If you're here reading this, you're already on your way, and I commend you for that. The advice I want to give you is this: be honest with yourself.

As a therapist with years of experience, I have seen countless individuals struggle with the same issue: they try to hide or romanticize their reality, thinking that it will make things easier or less painful. But the truth is that this approach only delays the healing process and prevents us from achieving true progress.

It's easy to think that being honest with ourselves means being harsh or critical, but that couldn't be further from the truth. Honesty is about acknowledging our thoughts, feelings, and behaviors, both the good and the bad, without judgment. It's about accepting our flaws and weaknesses while also recognizing our strengths and accomplishments. It's about being real with ourselves and others, no matter how difficult that may be.

At the entrance of the Temple of Delphi in ancient Greece, there was an inscription that read "Know thyself." It may seem like a simple concept, but it's one that has been echoed throughout history, across cultures and traditions. And for good reason: self-awareness is the key to unlocking our full potential.

One of the most powerful tools for developing self-awareness is journaling. By writing down our thoughts, feelings, and experiences, we gain clarity and insight into our inner world. We start to recognize patterns and triggers, and we can identify the areas of our lives that need attention and healing. And the best part? You don't need any special training or equipment to start journaling. All you need is a pen and paper (or a digital device) and a willingness to be honest with yourself.

As you begin your journaling practice, remember that the goal is not to be perfect or to have all the answers. It's simply to start a conversation with yourself and to listen to what you have to say. Give yourself permission to be vulnerable, to explore your feelings without judgment, and to ask yourself the hard questions. And above all, be patient and compassionate with yourself. This is a journey, and it takes time and effort to develop the skill of self-awareness.

But the rewards are worth it. By being honest with ourselves, we can live more authentic and fulfilling lives. We can make better decisions, build stronger relationships, and cultivate a deeper sense of purpose and meaning. We can free ourselves from the limiting beliefs and self-imposed barriers that hold us back, and we can step into our power as the creators of our own lives.

So, my friend, I urge you to take this advice to heart. Be honest with yourself, and watch as the world opens up before you. The possibilities are endless, and the only limit is the one you set for yourself.

<u>You</u>

Now ending this book, I am filled with a deep sense of gratitude for the opportunity to share my knowledge and experience with you, my dear reader. It is my hope that the information and insights contained within these pages will serve to inspire and empower you on your journey towards greater health and well-being.

As we have already discussed, Bach Flower Remedies have a rich history and a long tradition of use in promoting physical, emotional, and spiritual healing. They are a safe and natural alternative to conventional medicine, and can be used in conjunction with other therapies to achieve optimal health and wellness.

Throughout the course of this book, we have explored each of the 38 Flower Remedies in depth, discussing their individual properties, indications, and modes of use. We have also examined the principles and philosophy behind this powerful healing modality, and have learned how to select and administer remedies based on our own unique needs and circumstances.

But the true beauty of Bach Flower Remedies lies not only in their effectiveness, but in the deep sense of connection and empathy they can foster between ourselves and the natural world. By working with these remedies, we are invited to tune into the subtle energies and healing powers of the plants and flowers around us, and to develop a greater awareness of our own inner landscapes and emotional states.

So, as I dedicate this book to you, I do so with the utmost sincerity and reverence for the transformative power of Bach Flower Remedies. May it serve as a source of inspiration and guidance as you continue on your journey towards greater health, happiness, and wholeness. And may it remind you always of the infinite potential for healing and growth that resides within you, waiting to be unlocked and unleashed.

<u>*Final Notes:*</u>

I dedicate this book to my parents. To my siblings, Fabio and Denise, and their descendants, my beloved nieces and nephews, in order of arrival into this world: Eduardo, Bianca, Mellanie, Sophia, and Nicholas. And to Kerlinton, who has integrated so well into our family.

I also dedicate this book to a few special people: Lourdinha and Antonieta – friends, sisters of the path, mentors. And to the beloved ones who have passed and those who are still with us. Some of whom, without whom I would not be who I am: Sollon and Dr. Tsui – the best friends a person could have.

To you who have arrived here, I dedicate not only this book but also my deepest and most positive vibrations. Be happy.

In this Edition I reformatted the text to make it more visually appealing, although this caused the number of pages to increase and subsequently the final cost of the book. I removed the Table of Contents and added a section about the author, as I received a message requesting this information.

About the Author

Meet William Camolesi Di Biasi! He grew up in a family of teachers who instilled in him a love for learning and books since he was a kid. He spent his childhood surrounded by literature in a small town in the interior of Goias. As he got older, he moved to the capital city, Goiania, to pursue his passion for psychology.

Working for several years as a teacher. During that time, he became interested in alternative therapies and discovered his true passion for Holistic Therapy, which became his profession.

Writing has always been a passion, and he even participated in writing competitions in his city when he was young. He is also a member of the Society of Alternative Studies and trained as an acupuncturist at Unisaúde IPGU.

Believes in universalism and thinks that diverse philosophical perspectives can benefit humanity. Although he is a priest in his religious path, he believes that faith should not be labelled, and prejudice in any form is a scourge on humanity.

Outside of his professional pursuits, William is a loving son, brother, and uncle. He values simplicity in life and often practices yoga, tai chi, and other activities that connect him with nature and promote inner peace. His biggest dream is to become a father someday.

William Camolesi Di Biasi
camolesidibiasi@gmail.com

Thank You for Help me Grow!